Geriatric Medicine for Old Age Psychiatrists

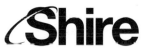

Geriatric Medicine for Old Age Psychiatrists

Alistair Burns
Head of Division of Psychiatry, Professor of Old Age Psychiatry
Education & Research Centre, Wythenshawe Hospital
Manchester, UK

Michael A Horan
Professor of Geriatric Medicine
University of Manchester,
Division of Medicine and Neuroscience, Hope Hospital, Salford
Consulting Physician to the David Lewis National Epilepsy Centre
Alderley Edge, UK

John F. Clague
Consultant Physician, Department of Medicine for the Elderly
University Hospital Aintree
Liverpool, UK

Gillian McLean
Consultant Psychiatrist for the Elderly
Falkirk and District Royal Infirmary
Falkirk, Scotland, UK

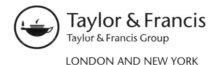

Taylor & Francis
Taylor & Francis Group

LONDON AND NEW YORK

First published in the United Kingdom in 2006
by Taylor & Francis,
an imprint of the Taylor & Francis Group,
2 Park Square, Milton Park
Abingdon, Oxon OX14 4RN, UK

Tel.:   +44 (0) 20 7017 6000
Fax.:   +44 (0) 20 7017 6699
E-mail: info.medicine@tandf.co.uk
Website: http://www.tandf.co.uk/medicine

British Library Cataloguing in Publication Data

Data available on application

Library of Congress Cataloging-in-Publication Data

Data available on application

ISBN10: 1-84184-393-8
ISBN13: 9-78-1-84184-393-3

Distributed in North and South America by

Taylor & Francis
2000 NW Corporate Blvd
Boca Raton, FL 33431, USA

Within Continental USA
Tel.: 800 272 7737; Fax.: 800 374 3401
Outside Continental USA
Tel.: 561 994 0555; Fax.: 561 361 6018
E-mail: orders@crcpress.com

Distributed in the rest of the world by
Thomson Publishing Services
Cheriton House
North Way
Andover, Hampshire SP10 5BE, UK
Tel.: +44 (0) 1264 332424
E-mail: salesorder.tandf@thomsonpublishingservices.co.uk

Composition by Parthenon Publishing
Printed and bound by Antony Rowe Ltd., Chippenham, Wiltshire, UK

Contents

List of contributors   vii

Preface   ix

1.   Introduction   1

2.   History and physical examination   9

3.   Interpretation of abnormal results   27

4.   Clinical management   55

5.   Clinical vignettes   205

6.   Commonly prescribed drugs   215

7.   Further reading   247

8.   Appendix   249

     Index   251

List of contributors

Alistair Burns MD, FRCP, FRCPsych, MPhil
Head of Division of Psychiatry
Professor of Old Age Psychiatry
Room PBS 18
Second Floor
Education and Research Centre
Wythenshawe Hospital
Manchester M23 9LT
UK

John E Clague MD, FRCP
Consultant Physician
Department of Medicine for the Elderly
University Hospital Aintree
Lower Lane
Liverpool L9 7AL
UK

Michael A Horan MA, MB, PhD, FRCP
Professor of Geriatric Medicine
University of Manchester
Clinical Sciences Building
Hope Hospital
Stott Lane
Salford M6 8HD
UK

Gillian McLean BSc(Hon), MBChB, DRCOG, MRCPsych
Consultant Psychiatrist for the Elderly
Department of Old Age Psychiatry
Falkirk & District Royal Infirmary
Majors Loan
Falkirk FK1 5QE
UK

Preface

The interface between physical ill health and mental health problems is complex. It is well recognised that there can often be primarily a psychiatric presentation of an underlying physical disease. The prevalence of the major psychiatric disorders (delirium, depression, dementia) is higher in people who are physically ill.

The reasoning behind this book is that it should serve as an update for practitioners in old age psychiatry who may not have had much exposure to general medical issues and that exposure may have been some while ago, with skills atrophying and knowledge waning over time.

We hope to summarise some of the major clinical problems seen not uncommonly in the general practice of old age psychiatry, review the process of history taking and examination in relation to physical health, try to help with the interpretation of investigations and provide a summary of some of the commoner drugs used.

It is not meant to replace the generally very cordial relations between colleagues in old age psychiatry and geriatric medicine, but perhaps more to give clinicians in the former discipline some confidence in what they are doing, and if it cuts out some unnecessary referrals or makes the information which backs up those referrals a little better, then the book will have been a success.

Alistair Burns
Michael Horan
John Clague
Gillian McLean

Introduction

MEDICINE IN OLD AGE

The practice of old age psychiatry differs from general adult psychiatry, not least because of the particular attributes of the patients presenting with psychiatric disorders. The most obvious difference is that the patients are old and will be well advanced along the trajectory of numerous age-related changes. Aging processes, at least in the biological sense, are relatively benign and are seldom manifested in the absence of some additional stressor. Indeed, we can usefully consider aging to be a progressive erosion of reserve capacities and an increased susceptibility to the effects of external stressors. As a rule of thumb, those under the age of 70 years will be physiologically similar to middle-aged people, whereas those over 75 years will show an increasing likelihood of age-related impairments.

Whether we consider it to be age-related or simply time-related, older people are also characterised by the accumulation of various, usually chronic, diseases. This phenomenon is often referred to as *co-morbidity* (or less accurately as *multiple pathology*) and is highly characteristic of older people. These co-morbid factors may have significant health and survival implications in their own right, but they will also frequently complicate the assessment and/or management of older people presenting with psychiatric disorders. In some instances, such as delirium, the psychiatric disorder may be a very direct consequence of the underlying physical disturbance. Thus, any practitioner in old age psychiatry must have a working knowledge of aging physiology, how drug handling and drug actions change in old age and the common somatic disorders of older people. They need to know what they can reasonably manage without the help of a physician (or sometimes, a surgeon) and also what is foolhardy for them to attempt to treat without such help. The following chapters are concerned with understanding the relevant physiology and the management of common medical problems. Where appropriate, guidance is given about how to treat these medical conditions; where inappropriate, we also suggest what information a physician or surgeon may want in order to make an assessment.

THE PRESENTATION OF DISEASE IN OLD AGE

The classical presentations of diseases given in popular textbooks will certainly be encountered in the medicine of old age. Some old people with a myocardial infarction do have crushing central chest pain radiating to the neck and arm and associated with nausea and vomiting (but not always!). However, less clear-cut presentations of many diseases are the rule rather than the exception. Four general modes of presentation can easily be recognised:

(1)   Typical;

(2)   Atypical;

(3)   Silent;

(4)   Pseudo-silent.

Descriptions of typical (classical) presentations can be found in any standard medical textbook and are not described further here.

Atypical presentations generally arise from interactions between aging and co-morbid factors, so that dysfunction in one organ or system can give rise to the dominant presenting symptoms and signs being manifestations of dysfunction in some other organ or system. Thus, delirium can be the presenting feature of almost any disease or disorder in older people. Some presentations are so common as to account for the majority of the clinical practice of most geriatricians. One of our great geriatricians, Bernard Isaacs, referred to them as the five 'I's':

(1)   Immobility (reduced activity and functional ability);

(2)   Instability (falls);

(3)   Insanity (delirium);

(4)   Incontinence;

(5)   Iatrogenic (caused by something a doctor has given).

To these, Kane has added a lot more 'I's' of geriatric medicine (see Table 1.1).

These atypical presentations can be extremely challenging to sort out, and demanding of considerable experience and diagnostic acumen.

Silent presentations are rather less common than typical and atypical ones, but they do occur. Very often, the patient is 'not right', 'unwell' or 'not

Table 1.1 The 'I's' of geriatric medicine

Immobility	Irritable colon
Instability	Isolation
Incontinence	Inanition (wasting)
Insanity	Impecunity (poverty)
Iatrogenic	Insomnia
Infection	Immune deficiency (controversial)
Impaired vision and hearing	Impotence

themselves', or has taken to bed. Beware especially the patient who says that they are about to die: it is not unusual for them then to do so (most often of a pulmonary embolus or massive haemorrhage). Silent presentations can be even more challenging to the doctor than atypical ones.

Pseudo-silent presentations are all too common: they represent a failure! They arise because a doctor is too inexperienced, lacks the necessary knowledge, gives up because it is just too difficult or simply can not be bothered. We provide you with enough information in the following chapters to avoid this trap. To paraphrase Einstein, 'Everything will be made as simple as possible, but not one bit simpler.'

THE MEDICAL APPROACH: THE CAREFUL DOCTOR

Most experienced physicians do not follow the logical standard we all learned in medical school: they tend to rely on wide experience and a good memory from which they have constructed patterns or templates against which they apply new pieces of information as they emerge. The subsequent approach is to seek further information to confirm or refute possible diagnoses. This approach is both effective and efficient, although it sometimes gets the diagnosis spectacularly wrong. Do not be surprised when an experienced physician solves a problem in a few minutes that you have grappled with for days (or longer): that is what he (she) is trained to do. Experienced surgeons are similarly capable. This is well illustrated by an anecdote about Walter Edward Dandy, an American pioneer of neurosurgery of Lancashire parents. He reviewed a patient, already anaesthetised, whose diagnosis had puzzled several of the physicians. Dandy immediately recommended a right-sided trepanation to drain the so-far undiagnosed brain abscess that he thought was producing the symptoms. As the pus drained, an amazed observer asked Dandy how he made the diagnosis and knew where to drill the trephining hole. Dandy replied 'God must have whispered in my ear.'

This approach works for the management of problems too, just as it does for diagnosis. Most experienced physicians know what is likely to happen if a particular treatment is given and how long it might take before it happens, so they have an intuitive grasp of when something is not quite right, which prompts a re-evaluation of the patient. We can not teach you this sort of experience, but we can present some general rules to avoid getting into difficulties worse than the presenting problem.

SOME GOLDEN RULES

Diagnosis

Always check some critical piece of information before acting on it. For example, check the blood pressure measurement yourself. Look at the 'sweat rash' reported by the nurse who is asking you to prescribe Canesten® or Timodine®: it may be, for example, a squamous carcinoma which will respond much better to surgery or radiotherapy. What you are told is a sacral pressure sore may actually turn out to be perianal Paget's disease, lichen sclerosus or Crohn's disease. Do not blindly accept the interpretation that someone had an epileptic seizure: get a description of exactly what happened. Some words, such as collapse, do not have any precise meaning: it can refer to a fall, presyncope or unconsciousness: always check what the informant means.

Investigation

Investigations should generally be used to test diagnostic hypotheses and not to generate them. However, screening investigations do have a role in the medicine of old age. However, be aware that if you perform enough tests, you will eventually find one or more that falls outside the normal range, and you will then have orphan data in search of a hypothesis. One wag defined a normal person as one who has not been sufficiently investigated. We would suggest the screening tests listed in Table 1.2 as suitable for this purpose when you encounter a new patient. These tests need doing only once: other tests or repeats should be performed only to answer specific questions. If you do request any investigations, you *must* look at the results. Any urgent radiographs must be sent for reporting by a radiologist.

The first question you should ask yourself is whether or not you know how to interpret the tests you are requesting. If you do not know, you should either find out or not perform the test. Even if you do know how to interpret a test, you do not necessarily have to perform it. Apart from the one-off screening tests suggested, you should ask the following questions:

Table 1.2 Suitable screening tests

Full blood count (FBC)

Biochemical profile
      urea and electrolytes
      glucose
      liver function tests
      albumin and globulins
      calcium

Thyroid function tests
      T_3
      T_4
      TSH*

Blood lipids (optional)

ESR (but difficult to interpret)

Urine stick testing (including blood, protein and nitrite)

Some psychiatrists recommend the following tests in the setting of cognitive impairment, although there is little evidence to support this:

Vitamin B_{12}

Folic acid

Syphilis serology

---

* Some laboratories measure only thyroid-stimulating hormone (TSH) for the purpose of screening; T_3, tri-iodothyronine; T_4, thyroxine; ESR, erythrocyte sedimentation rate

(1)   What will you do if the test is positive?

(2)   What will you do if the test is negative?

If the answer to these two questions is the same, there is no indication to perform the test.

Prescribing (see Chapter 6)

Before prescribing a drug, decide what you expect the drug to do. Also, set a time when you will review whether or not it has done this. If your goal has not been achieved, it is most likely that the diagnosis was wrong or you have selected the wrong treatment. Whatever the explanation, you must seek it.

If you prescribe a drug, you *must* know what side-effects the drug might have and any important interactions. Later in the book, we address the topic of therapeutics in more detail, and we summarise common side-effects of the most frequently used drugs. When you are prescribing, try to stick to the drugs that you know and you will prescribe them safely. Also, make sure that you are aware of any local guidelines and policies relating to problems you commonly encounter. If you must prescribe a drug that you do not know, ensure that you check an up-to-date copy of the *British National Formulary* (BNF) for important side-effects, interactions and any dose adjustments recommended for older patients.

Get into the habit of reviewing drug charts regularly. What is the indication for each of the drugs? Anticonvulsants and antidepressants have uses other than their main ones (pain, for example). Are all the drugs still indicated? Could the problem that you are addressing at the moment be caused by a drug or drug interaction? Have the prescribed drugs actually been given to the patient and has the patient subsequently ingested them? Never increase the dose of a drug without being sure that the previously prescribed dose has been given and ingested!

Management

Many older people will already have multiple diagnoses and some of them may not be well established, or they may even be wrong. Diagnosing a condition does not necessarily mean that it needs treatment. Most people taking more than seven drugs will have new problems caused by the drugs (or interactions), and they will probably not be taking them as prescribed in any case. However, we have encountered one patient taking 38 different medications, some for the side-effects of already prescribed drugs. Regrettably, she was taking them *all* exactly as prescribed: her husband had taken early retirement to supervise the medication schedule. The drugs killed her!

Most practitioners of medicine in old age are more concerned with problems and problem management rather than simply with diagnoses. For both investigation and treatment, list the problems and consider which are stable/unstable, active/inactive. Consider which are the most straightforward and most troublesome and concentrate on those. Worry about the remaining ones at some other time, but *do not* forget about them.

Loeb's Laws (points 1–3 below) probably constitute the most sensible advice for practicing medicine:

(1)   If what you are doing is working, carry on;

(2)   If it is not working, stop;

(3)   If you do not know what to do, do not do anything (*other than seek help*);

(4)   Do not try to be too clever (our addition).

Most patients will have simple, straightforward things wrong with them and not rare conditions. Learn the common disorders and then you will know when something does not quite fit. You can then look it up or seek help. Trying to be too clever can get you into trouble. Most doctors will not see more than one case of infective endocarditis during an entire professional lifetime; they will see lots of respiratory infections, urine infections and skin infections. Rare presentations of common conditions are much more common than rare disorders, even common presentations of rare conditions. However hard we try, we will make more misdiagnoses of obturator hernia than correct ones, mainly because the prior probability of this diagnosis is low. You will only recognise what you know, so make sure you know the common things.

2   History and physical examination

THE BASIC MEDICAL HISTORY

You will be seeing patients whose primary problems are psychiatric ones. However, always remember to check whether the patient has any other problems that they think you need to know about. If the patient volunteers any, you need to ask further detailed questions about them. Thereafter, screening questions will uncover problems in the major organs and systems. Table 2.1 gives a list of useful questions organised around function. This is an approach used by one of us when screening patients in the orthopedics and trauma wards: it not only uncovers problems but also indicates how severe the problem is and how it impacts on someone's life. When positive answers are found, clarification and relevant physical examination are essential. For those who prefer to follow a more traditional approach, we have listed suitable organ-system-related questions in Table 2.2.

THE BASIC MEDICAL EXAMINATION

A detailed physical examination is time-consuming and demanding of considerable skill and experience. If you read books on physical examination, you may well be overwhelmed by the number of physical signs described there. Curiously, aspects of physical examination have not been subjected to the same level of scrutiny as have other aspects of medical practice: many aspects of physical examination are not very reproducible and have low inter-rater reliability. We try to address only those physical signs that are straightforward to perform and have proven clinical utility and reproducibility.

We have also considered the context in which the physical examination will be done – perhaps with fully clothed patients for whom undressing is not always very practical. This situation is certainly *not* ideal. Thus, we have tried to suggest things that maximise the amount of useful information to be collected with the minimum of effort in a patient whose neck, arms and legs (below the knees) can be readily exposed and in whom the abdomen is

Table 2.1 The medical history – a functional approach

(1) Any problems with washing/dressing/preparing food?
Musculoskeletal
Neurological
Cardiovascular
Respiratory
Visual

(2) Any problems eating/drinking?
Musculoskeletal
Neurological
Visual
Oral conditions
Gastrointestinal

(3) Any problems getting around inside?
Musculoskeletal
Neurological
Cardiovascular
Respiratory
Visual

(4) Any problems reading/watching TV/listening to the radio?
Musculoskeletal
Neurological
Visual
Auditory

(5) Any problems getting around outside?
Musculoskeletal
Neurological
Cardiovascular
Respiratory
Visual
Continence

(6) Have you stopped doing things you really enjoy?
Musculoskeletal

continued

Table 2.1 (*continued*)

    Neurological
    Cardiovascular
    Respiratory
    Visual
    Continence

(7)   Sleeping?
    Musculoskeletal
    Cardiovascular
    Respiratory
    Bladder

(8)   Do you have pain anywhere?
    Musculoskeletal
    Neurological
    Gastrointestinal
    Urogenital

(9)   How many falls in the last 6 months?
    Musculoskeletal
    Neurological
    Cardiovascular

(10) What medicines (including over-the-counter) are you taking?

---

accessible. Clearly, if the patient volunteers specific problems or you uncover them during history-taking or during a basic examination, more detailed examination is mandatory and the relevant body part(s) must be properly exposed. Table 2.3 summarises what we think is useful and practical for routine physical examination in the setting of an old age psychiatry service.

GENERAL APPEARANCE

The general appearance of a patient can be quite revealing. Does the patient appear well or unwell, neat or unkempt, fat or thin, in discomfort or breathless? If the patient appears to be wasted, a full, detailed physical

Table 2.2 The medical history – a traditional approach

Respiratory
Cough
Sputum
Haemoptysis
Wheeze
Shortness of breath

Cardiovascular
Orthopnoea
Chest pain
Paroxysmal nocturnal dyspnoea
Ankle swelling
Palpitations

Alimentary
Appetite
Weight loss
Swallowing problems
Dysphagia
Nausea
Abdominal pain
Vomiting
Haematemesis
Melaena
Rectal bleeding
Altered bowel habit

Neurological
Headaches
Tinnitus
Diplopia
Loss of consciousness
Balance
Weakness
Numbness

Sphincter control
Vision
Hearing

Musculoskeletal
Joint pain
Stiffness
Joints give way

Skin
Rashes
Sores/ulcers

Urogenital (men)
Frequency
Nocturia
Dysuria
Haematuria
Stream
Erectile problems
Continence

Urogenital (women)
Frequency
Nocturia
Dysuria
Haematuria
Postmenopausal bleeding
Vaginal discharge
Continence

List of medications

Family history
Parents
Siblings

Table 2.3 The basic physical examination

General appearance

Weight

Face
  asymmetry
  rashes/bruising
  lumps (feel for nodes)
  ears (tophi)

Mouth
  angular cheilosis (perlèche)
  oral hygiene
  moist/dry (dehydration,
    medications, Sjögren's
    syndrome)
  teeth
  tongue (smooth with burning
    suggests vitamin B deficiency)

Vision
  near (reading)
  distant (describing something
    over 10 metres away)
  ophthalmoscope if visual
    impairment – look for
    cataracts
  visual fields (hemianopia)

Otoscopy (if hearing decreased –
  look for wax)

Neck bruits

Pulse (rate and rhythm)

Blood pressure – sitting (lying, and
  standing if there is any suggestion
  of syncope)

Hands
  tar stains from smoking
  joint disease
  clubbing
  manipulation of small objects

Abdomen
  masses
  bruits

Leg
  oedema
  popliteal pulse
  brown pigmentation
  lipodermatosclerosis
  ulceration
  tendon reflexes

Ankles/feet
  swelling
  dorsalis pedis and posterior
    tibial artery pulses
  digital gangrene
  callus
  ulcers
  deformity
  nails
  tendon reflexes
  light touch
  pain sensation
  joint position sense
  plantar responses

examination will be needed: depression and dementia are not the only causes of weight loss. Is there a smell? We have listed some characteristic smells
in Table 2.4 as they occasionally point the doctor in the right direction.
Look at the face and head for symmetry (facial weakness, Paget's disease of
bone), rashes, basal cell carcinoma in the nasolabial furrow or near the eye,
bruising (falls), lumps (parotid tumours, enlarged lymph nodes), hair (myxoedema) and ears (tophi, squamous carcinoma).

Head and neck

Next look at the lips, mouth and tongue. Angular cheilosis suggests deficiency of iron, folate, B vitamins or diabetes mellitus with candidiasis. Inside
the mouth, oral hygiene will be apparent. Is the mouth dry or moist (hydration state, medications and Sjögren's syndrome)? Dribbling saliva is common in advanced Parkinson's disease or after a stroke. Look at the teeth and
consider dental referral, if indicated. Look at the tongue for deviation, fasciculation, texture and appearance. A smooth tongue (often with a burning

Table 2.4 Characteristic smells

What you smell	*What it may mean*
Alcohol	alcohol use/abuse
Ammonia	urinary incontinence
	uraemia
Faeces	poor hygiene
	faecal incontinence
	leg ulcer, pressure ulcer
	anaerobic infection
Halitosis	dental problems
	poor oral hygiene
	sinusitis
	gastric malignancy
Tobacco*	smoking

*Most important in clinical practice

sensation) suggests vitamin B deficiency. A blue tongue suggests central cyanosis. Are there any red or white patches on the tongue or elsewhere in the mouth (*Candida*, leukoplakia, erythroplakia, lichen planus)? Are there any lumps or ulcers (oral cancer is mainly a disease of the old)? Assess tongue movements: you should already be aware of dysarthria, if present. If the voice is hoarse, there may be vocal cord paralysis: you will need to examine the chest and request a chest radiograph.

Next, look at the eyes. Do they appear symmetrical? Do the eyelids droop? Is the conjunctiva inflamed or unusually pale? Is there an ectropion or an entropion? Is the sclera white, red or yellow? Check near vision by getting the patient to read something. Check distance vision by having the patient describe something > 10m away. Check visual fields (hemianopia): this can be done conveniently by holding up a piece of string horizontally and asking the patient to touch the middle. Patients with a hemianopia indicate the midpoint of the intact field of view which will appear eccentrically placed to the examiner. If there is visual impairment, the lens and retina should be examined. An ophthalmoscope is a difficult instrument to use: ophthalmologists hardly ever use it other than as a light source. The easiest disorder to detect is cataract (impaired red reflex). Examining the retina is much more difficult, especially in older people with small pupils; if you do not know how to interpret what you find, there is little point to dilating the pupils. If there is evidence of a hearing impairment, this is a good time to examine the ear with an otoscope (mainly to look for ear wax, foreign bodies or perforations of the ear drum). Next, examine the neck. You should at least check for carotid bruits and enlarged lymph nodes. Remember, absence of carotid bruits does not rule out significant carotid artery atheroma. Assessing the jugular venous pressure is not easy, and to enable you to do it properly, the patient must be undressed and in the correct position.

Thorax and abdomen

Examining the heart and lungs requires the patient to be undressed, and you may not feel comfortable in the interpretation of heart sounds and murmurs anyway. If you find any enlarged lymph nodes, you will need to examine the chest and abdomen with the patient undressed, and also request a chest radiograph. Even if the patient is dressed and sitting in a chair, try to feel the abdomen for an aortic aneurysm: an expansile mass may be felt and there may be an abdominal bruit.

Upper limbs

Next move to the arms, which need to be exposed sufficiently for you to measure the blood pressure: do this yourself and do not rely on the chart. Arms greater than 27 cm circumference indicate the need for a cuff larger than the standard one to avoid overestimating the true blood pressure. If there is a history of any 'funny turns' or blackouts, check the blood pressure in *both* arms (subclavian steal syndrome). In the presence of atrial fibrillation, blood pressure measurements will be inaccurate unless a special technique is used (not described here). Check the pulse rate and rhythm. Look for evidence of joint disease and tophi. Bruising at this location is common, and comes about after minor trauma to thin skin with fragile blood vessels (senile purpura). Feel around the elbow for rheumatoid nodules. Check the upper limb tendon reflexes. Detailed sensory testing is not necessary, but check for gross sensory loss or sensory inattention. Check for upper-limb ataxia with the finger–nose test. Truncal ataxia will already have been assessed by watching the patient's ability to sit upright, unsupported, on a chair. A useful screen for sensory and motor impairments as well as joint malfunction is to ask the patient to try to scratch his/her back between the shoulder blades, using each arm in turn, and to manipulate small objects with the hands (e.g. undo and fasten a button). Test muscle strength at the shoulder (abduction) and observe the arm for fasciculations. Observe for abnormal movements at rest, while sustaining a fixed posture and during movement.

Inspect the fingers. Tar stains indicate tobacco smoking. Evidence of osteoarthritis, rheumatoid disease or gout should be readily apparent. Test muscle strength (finger spreading). Are the palmar creases pale (anaemia)? Is there a tremor (most likely Parkinson's disease, anxiety, essential tremor or thyrotoxicosis)? Look at the nails for clubbing. Nail colour may point to diagnoses: blue suggests cyanosis, red suggests polycythaemia, white suggests hypoalbuminaemia and half-and-half nails suggest uraemia, liver disease or osteoporosis. Faecal contamination of the hands and nails in cognitively impaired patients is highly suggestive of faecal loading, with repeated attempts at auto-evacuation with the fingers.

Lower limbs

Now move down to the lower leg and look for oedema and ulceration. Observe for abnormal movements (especially akathisia and myoclonus). Check the tendon reflexes and plantar responses. Check for gross sensory impairment, as for the upper limbs. In addition, check light touch, pain and position sensation in the big toe. Check muscle strength (hip flexion and ankle dorsiflexion). The general state of the feet should be obvious and the help of a podiatrist may be needed: foot disorders are common in old people, impair many aspects of function and are often overlooked. Table 2.5 lists some common foot disorders of older people.

Finally, before you finish, you need to check gait and balance: simple screening tests such as the 'get-up-and-go' test and the Romberg test will usually suffice. These tests are described in Table 2.6. Abnormal findings will prompt a more detailed examination and referral to a geriatrician for further assessment.

Table 2.5 Common foot disorders of the elderly

Biomechanical
hallux valgus

Painful keratoses and corns

Skin and nails
dry skin
oedema
ulcers (venous, arterial, diabetic, pressure)
onychauxis (thickened nails)
onychogryphosis (overgrown, deformed, thickened nails)
tinea pedis (fungal infection, usually between toes)

Joint disease
osteoarthritis
rheumatoid disease
gout

Arterial insufficiency
may cause gangrene and ulceration

Tumours
squamous carcinoma
basal cell carcinoma (occasionally)

Table 2.6 Gait and balance assessment

---

(1) 'Get up and go' test

There are many variations of this test. It is used in ambulatory patients only and a single practice run is permitted. Usual walking aids may be used.

Stand from a high-seated, straight-backed chair with arm rests;

Stand for 10 seconds;

Walk 3 metres;

Turn;

Walk back to the chair;

Sit down again.

Watch the patient perform each component and assess the ease, accuracy and safety of each component.

(2) Romberg test

Ask the patient to stand with the feet apart, and then bring the feet together. A normal response is being able to stand with the feet together. Minor imbalance without falling is acceptable. Marked imbalance, particularly if the person is likely to fall, suggests ataxia. If stance is normal, as tested above, get the patient to extend the arms to 90° and to close his or her eyes. A normal person can do this without undue foot movements or sway. Unilateral sway suggests an ipsilateral cerebellar lesion. Bilateral sway indicates ataxia of some sort.

THE NEUROLOGICAL EXAMINATION

Old age psychiatrists are predominantly involved with disorders of the brain, so it is essential that you can perform a competent neurological examination and be able to interpret what you find. However, you are not expected to be able to achieve the same level of competence as a neurologist. For your convenience, we have included in the Appendix the scheme for the general neurological examination that one of us uses when assessing such patients. For patients suspected to have dementia, you will need to concentrate on those aspects that help you diagnose the likely subtype. In

Table 2.7 The neurological examination in dementia

Ataxia	*Akinesia/rigidity*
Alcohol	Lewy body disease
Thiamine deficiency	Alzheimer's disease
Spinocerebellar degeneration	Progressive supranuclear palsy
Hydrocephalus	Huntington's disease
vCJD	Corticobasal degeneration
Multiple sclerosis	CJD
	Heavy-metal poisoning
Focal signs	Traumatic encephalopathy
Vascular dementia	(dementia pugilistica)
Brain tumour	
Brain infiltration	*Neuropathy*
Haematoma	Vascular dementia (diabetes)
CJD	Alcohol
Motor neuron disease	Vasculitis
	Uraemic encephalopathy
Myoclonus	Paraneoplastic disorder
Alzheimer's disease	
CJD	
AIDS dementia	
Metabolic encephalopathy	

vCJD, variant Creutzfeldt–Jakob disease; AIDS, acquired immune deficiency syndrome

the main, you will be seeking localising (hard) and semi- or non-localising (soft) signs. These signs, in the setting of a likely dementia, point the way to the likely diagnosis (diagnoses) and will help in the choice of further investigations. We summarise some of these in Table 2.7.

LEGAL ASPECTS OF TREATING MEDICAL CONDITIONS IN THE MENTALLY ILL

There are several factors that are relevant to all of your clinical practice:

(1)   You owe a duty of care to anyone that you accept as a patient, but not to those who are not your patients.

(2)   You have no doctor–patient relationship with the relatives of your patient.

(3)   You must act in accordance with a practice accepted as proper by a responsible body of doctors.

(4)   Departure from accepted practice does not *automatically* constitute negligence.

(5)   The standard of care expected may be lower in an emergency.

Thus, in cases of negligence litigation, a duty of care must first be established. Thereafter, a breach of that duty must be demonstrated to have led to the adverse consequence (harm), which could reasonably have been avoided.

All medical activity is potentially a trespass against the person and, therefore, consent is required. A patient who is not competent to give consent is unable to legitimise medical treatment, even if they voluntarily agree to it. Assault is a threat of violence that induces fear: battery is an actual bodily contact. Unconsented touching of a patient lacking the necessary capacity to give consent would be defended as a justifiable wrong.

In the National Health Service (NHS), any claim would be against the relevant health body (usually the Trust); in principle, the Trust could seek to recover its losses from you, its 'wrongful servant', although this is very unlikely. If the wrong is more serious, it may become a criminal matter, and the charge is likely to be actual bodily harm (ABH) or grievous bodily harm (GBH). If death ensues, the charge would be manslaughter or murder. Criminal charges more often arise from acts of omission than of commission. Liability under the criminal law is personal and you cannot be indemnified against it: any criminal conviction will be reported to the General Medical Council (GMC). Further, an employer cannot direct you to commit any act whatsoever that contravenes the criminal law.

The rights of a patient

There is no specific statute that provides patients with enforceable rights. The Patient's Charter has no legal force at all: it is simply something that the NHS should aspire to. However, the Human Rights Act (HRA) 1998 came into force in October 2000. It requires the Government to maintain and uphold the rights specified in the European Convention on Human

Rights (ECHR). Any emanation of the State or organ of Government has the same responsibilities as the Government itself, although this does not apply in the private health sector. This duty applies to you personally. Thus, any medical/therapeutic intervention might be regarded to contravene Article 3 of the Convention.

The major implications of the HRA for health-care are four-fold:

(1) Patients will be able to challenge public bodies in the domestic courts if their rights have been breached.

(2) Human rights issues may be raised in all medical litigation.

(3) Judicial scrutiny of decisions made by public bodies will become more rigorous and will focus on the rights of the individual rather than on the duties of the public body.

(4) All legislation must be read and given effect in a way which is compatible with Convention rights.

The ECHR rights most likely to be involved in medical practice are:

(1) Article 2* – The right to life;

(2) Article 3* – The right not to be subjected to torture, inhuman or degrading treatment;

(3) Article 8† – The right to private and family life;

(4) Article 9† – The right to freedom of thought, conscience and religion;

(5) Article 11† – The right to protection of health;

(6) Article 13* – The right to social and medical assistance;

(7) Article 14* – The right to enjoy Convention rights without discrimination.

(*Absolute rights; †qualified rights)

Consent

The right to consent is not extensive: a patient has a right to know what is to be done to them but not necessarily to know why it is to be done. If there was a right for the patient to know why, there would be a corresponding duty to tell, which might not always be in the patient's interests. The judgement, how much to tell about 'why', is a matter for the doctor. Thus, it is lawful to withhold information covered by the Data Protection Act (e.g. contents of the medical record) on the grounds that it may be harmful or unduly distressing. Be aware of your obligations under the Data Protection Act, as contraventions carry criminal penalties, not civil ones.

There is no notion of informed consent in British law, although there is in the USA. Informed consent requires that all information is given and every potential risk is explained. British law refers not to informed consent, but to 'valid' or 'effective' consent, which requires an explanation of the nature, purpose and likely outcome of the proposed intervention in broad terms. The binding legal principle relating to consent and the duty to disclose possibly adverse consequences comes from the well-known Siddaway case (1985). The level of risk that must be explained is in the order of 1–2%. The onus is on the patient to ask about lesser risks if he/she wants to know about them. If the patient does ask, a truthful answer must be given. Once consent has been given, it remains valid until the procedure is done or the consent is withdrawn, whichever is the sooner.

The equally well-known Chester (2004) case appears to override Siddaway, but the issue here masqueraded as a consent issue: it was actually an issue of causation. This case arose from a complication of back surgery which the patient averred she had not been told about, although if she had been told, she would probably still have had the surgery after thinking about it for a period of time. However, the House of Lords took the view that having the complication was a matter of chance: if the patient had undergone the surgery at a different time, she might not have got the complication and she was therefore entitled to damages. This too is a binding precedent that relates to causation, and raises interesting possibilities for complications arising after cancelled and rescheduled procedures.

Consent differs from mere submission: it must be freely and voluntarily given. You need to assess the patient's understanding of what they have been told. If a competent patient chooses to devolve the decision to you or to some other person, that is acceptable and you must record the fact clearly in the case notes. A signed consent form does not constitute consent, it is merely a record thereof, and it may not always be valid. The lack of a signed consent form does not necessarily mean that valid consent has not been given.

Consent to medical treatment in Scotland

The Adults with Incapacity (Scotland) Act 2000 sets out a framework for regulating affairs of adults who have impaired capacity. In the case of medical treatment and research, it provides a clear statutory framework regulating what may be done by medical practitioners and others acting with authority. 'Incapable' means incapable of acting, making decisions, communicating decisions, understanding decisions or retaining the memory of decisions in relation to any particular matter by reason of mental disorder or communication problems due to a physical disability. Anyone carrying out functions under the Act must apply the general principles of benefit, minimum intervention, taking account of adults wishes and feelings, consultation with relevant others and encouragement of the adult to exercise any residual capacity. Appointment of a 'proxy' (welfare attorney, a person authorised under an intervention order or welfare guardian) is strongly advised as there are requirements under Part 5 of the Act (Medical Treatment and Research) to involve such proxies in decision making about medical treatment and research.

Part 5 of the Act specifically gives authority to treat a patient who is incapable of consenting to the treatment in question, on the issuing of a certificate of incapacity. The general principles of the Act outlined above must still be applied. However the common law authority to treat a patient in an emergency situation still remains. Medical treatment is defined in the Act as 'any procedure or treatment designed to safeguard or promote physical or mental health'. Authority is obtained by completion of the certificate of incapacity and signed by the medical practitioner primarily responsible for carrying out the intervention. For people requiring multiple or complex healthcare interventions a treatment plan could be, but does not have to be, drawn up. No treatment plans can however be drawn up that would normally require the signed consent of the adult and a separate certificate of incapacity is required to be drawn up for each of these interventions, e.g. a surgical procedure. Consent of a proxy with welfare powers, where reasonable and practicable, should be sought. Names can be provided by contacting the Public Guardian who retains a register of such nominees. The duration of the certificate should relate to the expected duration of the treatment and the incapacity, but should not exceed one year. In some cases where a patient is unable due to incapacity to consent to treatment for a mental illness, the Act may be used. However if a patient actively refuses treatment for a mental health problem then they should be formally detained under the Mental Health Act in order that they might benefit from the additional protections that act offers. The Mental Health Act does not allow compulsory treatment for a medical disorder, and if the patient is deemed incapable of giving informed consent to such an intervention, then it may be necessary to invoke both acts.

It is best practice to proceed with treatment when there is a consensus of opinion. Where disputes between the medical practitioner and proxy arise, the Mental Welfare commission can request a further report from a nominated medical practitioner. If the two medical practitioners are in agreement then the treatment can progress without the consent of the proxy or continuing disputes can be referred to the Court of Session (www. scotland/govuk/justice/incapacity/, www. scotland-legislation.hmso.gov.uk/).

Capacity

In 1960, the English courts lost their *parens patriae* jurisdiction over the affairs of incompetent adults. This arose as a consequence of the Mental Health Act 1959 and revocation of the Warrant under the Sign Manual. Thus, in England, Wales and Northern Ireland, no adult can consent on behalf of another except under the circumstances of those detained under the Mental Health Act, which permits unconsented treatment of the *mental* disorder but not of any other disorder. The provisions of the Mental Health Act cannot be overridden by an advance directive. In Scotland, the law is different, and there are circumstances in which proxy consent is accepted as valid.

The law presumes that any adult has the capacity to consent, and the legal test of such capacity is currently that:

(1)   They understand the predicament in broad terms;

(2)   They appreciate the choices and their consequences in broad terms;

(3)   They can retain the information and reflect upon it;

(4)   They can communicate their choice in some way.

Hopefully, psychiatrists will be well used to the practicalities of assessing capacity.

When capacity is lacking, any medical intervention outside the narrow provisions of the Mental Health Act will be unlawful, and any treatment given must be under circumstances that the decision is defensible in order to protect the doctor from liability for battery. The circumstances of this are:

(1)   Emergency treatment to preserve life/limb (necessity);

(2)   Best interests (get colleagues to agree);

(3)   Apply to the Court for a declaration that it is not unlawful;

(4)   Discuss with the family;

(5)   Advance directive.

Advance directives must conform to all other requirements of consent, and they are only binding if they are clear and unambiguous and describe precisely the circumstances under which the decision must be made. Advance directives do not have to be in writing, but a written one is more certain.

The Mental Capacity Act 2005

Following a Law Commission Report (1995), the Government indicated its intention to legislate. The draft Mental Capacity Bill underwent a consultation exercise and was reported on by the Joint Scrutiny Committee (Session 2002-03). The report was considered by The Department for Constitutional Affairs and a revised Bill was published.

This proposed legislation received the Royal Assent in April 2005 but it is unlikely to come into force before 2007. It provides for a new "lasting power of attorney" that extends beyond the direction of property. The "attornee" is obliged to act in the patient's best interests but must respect any "advance refusal" that is specified. If a person lacking capacity has not made a lasting power of attorney, a relative can apply to the newly constituted Court of Protection to grant such a power. Advance directives are placed on a statutory basis and they are required to be written down unless they are communicated to the doctor during the course of treatment.

The new Court of Protection assumes the High Court's inherent jurisdiction and covers matters of property, finance, health and welfare and best interests remains the overriding principle. The Court can appoint Deputies possessing health and welfare powers. There will also be a duty on NHS bodies to seek advice from an "Independent Consultee" before providing serious medical treatment to an incapacitated person for whom no other person is in a position to speak (an unbefriended person).

Medicine at the end of life

The law makes a presumption in favour of life as a 'boon and a blessing', and the HRA confers a right to life. Care, as opposed to medical treatment, can never be lawfully withheld. However, recognising that death is imminent, it is part of good care to permit, or not prevent nature from taking its course. Food and fluids are at the interface between care (which must be given) and treatment (which need not be given). If it is contemplated to withhold food and fluids, the best interests test cannot apply because nobody is viewed to have an interest in death. Their withdrawal/withholding must be on the grounds of futility, intolerability, overriding risk or the presence of an advance directive related to tube feeding.

The legal position on the withdrawal of artificial nutrition and hydration (ANH) was recently considered in a controversial decision of Munby J in *R (on the application of Burke) v General Medical Council* [2004], which on appeal, in May 2005, was overturned. It is not clear whether or not the case will now go to the House of Lords. The issues are so important that the case is likely to go to the House of Lords. In this case, a patient suffering from cerebellar degeneration sought to challenge GMC guidance on the withdrawal of ANH by way of judicial review on the grounds of incompatibility with articles 2, 3, 6, 8 and 14 of the ECHR.

The judge considered the position of the competent patient, incompetent patient and advance directives. He reiterated the long-established proposition that the treatment decisions in relation to incompetent patients who have not made advance directives are to be determined by reference to 'best interests'. More particularly, he drew the distinction between those patients who are incurable, those who are terminally ill and those who are dying, drawing out that what is in the patients' 'best interests' may depend on the different stages of their illness. His judgement explored the tension between the sanctity of life, personal autonomy and human dignity both in common law and under the ECHR, and the inter-relationship between articles 2, 3 and 8 of the ECHR. Adopting reasoning in earlier cases, he confirmed that 'best interests' are not limited to 'best medical interests' but must be viewed more widely. Other than in exceptional circumstances or where the patient is dying, the starting point must be what he described as the very strong presumption in favour of taking all steps which prolong life, albeit that he recognised that where the patient is dying the goal may properly be to ease suffering rather than achieve a short prolongation of life. However, he held that where the patient is gravely disabled but not dying, then the assessment of 'best interests' has to be made from the patient's perspective; and where life-prolonging treatment is providing some benefit, it should be provided unless it is intolerable.

'Do not resuscitate' (DNR) orders are in fact simply recommendations, and are only valid at the moment they are made. When the event provoking a decision about resuscitation occurs, a new decision must be made. Superior orders may be a mitigating circumstance, but they are not a defence.

3   Interpretation of abnormal results

CALCIUM

Calcium has important metabolic, physiological and structural roles: more than 99% is in the bony skeleton. Of the daily dietary intake, 20–40% is absorbed, depending on the nature of the diet. About half of the circulating calcium exists in the ionised form, the rest being bound to albumin or complexed to other small molecules. It is the ionised calcium that is physiologically active and affects neuromuscular excitability and the release of parathyroid hormone. In the presence of acidosis, more calcium is ionised. Most of the 250 mmol or so of calcium filtered by the glomeruli each day is reabsorbed in the proximal convoluted tubule without hormonal regulation. Reabsorption of the remainder in the distal convoluted tubule is regulated by parathyroid hormone (PTH).

The plasma ionised calcium is the main regulator of PTH secretion, although magnesium is also involved. PTH stimulates osteoclasts to resorb bone and the cells of the distal nephron to absorb calcium. It also induces the enzyme complex in the nephron that converts 25-OH vitamin D to 1,25-$(OH)_2$ vitamin D, which stimulates calcium (and phosphate) absorption in the gut.

Other hormones influence calcium. Calcitonin, released from the parafollicular cells of the thyroid gland in response to a high concentration of ionised calcium, opposes bone resorption and increases the renal clearance of calcium and phosphate. Thyroid hormone tends to increase the rate of calcium resorption from bone. Glucocorticoids, particularly in therapeutic doses, reduce calcium absorption and increase calcium loss.

Most laboratories still measure total calcium and also report a value corrected for the prevailing albumin concentration. This is usually done by calculating the difference of the actual albumin concentration from 40 g/l and adding or subtracting 0.02 mmol/l for each gram difference (add for albumin levels < 40 g/l, and vice versa). Some laboratories report ionised calcium, for which no such adjustment is needed.

When interpreting abnormalities of calcium metabolism, it is necessary to have some other biochemical results routinely available:

(1)   Albumin;

(2)   Urea and creatinine;

(3)   Phosphate;

(4)   Alkaline phosphatase.

Hypercalcaemia

In the setting of an old age psychiatry service, over 90% of cases of hyper-calcaemia will very likely be explained by either primary hyperparathy-roidism or cancer (either metastatic or as a paraneoplastic phenomenon), although it may also be a complication of treatment with lithium. The high-er is the calcium concentration, the more likely it is that cancer is the cause. The presence of a low phosphate concentration suggests a raised PTH level.

Other causes of hypercalcaemia include:

(1)   Sarcoid;

(2)   Hypervitaminosis D;

(3)   Renal failure;

(4)   Thiazide diuretics;

(5)   Thyrotoxicosis;

(6)   Addison's disease;

(7)   Paget's disease of bone.

Mild hypercalcaemia may be asymptomatic, and discovered after sending blood for a biochemical profile. The more rapid is the rise and the higher is the calcium concentration, the more likely patients are to present with neuropsychiatric features: malaise, lethargy, muscle weakness, disorienta-tion, psychosis, drowsiness and coma are all encountered. Other symptoms include thirst, polyuria, anorexia, nausea, vomiting, abdominal pain and constipation.

All patients with hypercalcaemia require investigation and treatment, and therefore must be referred to a physician for this. Emergency treatment is not needed for a calcium concentration < 3.0 mmol/l; patients whose cal-cium concentration is > 3.2 mmol/l definitely do. Emergency treatment is initially with fluids to restore euvolaemia, after which the fluids are contin-ued and loop diuretics are added to promote urine losses. Thereafter, one of the second-line therapies may be needed (calcitonin, bisphosphonates, gallium nitrate, glucocorticoids, haemodialysis).

Hypocalcaemia

Hypocalcaemia is rare, and you are not likely to encounter it. It generally occurs in one of the following five settings:

(1)   Secondary hyperparathyroidism (patients with renal failure);

(2)   Post-thyroid/parathyroid surgery;

(3)   Autoimmune parathyroid failure;

(4)   Osteomalacia (vitamin D deficiency);

(5)   Magnesium deficiency.

Acutely, it causes circumoral tingling and tetany. It may also cause laryngospasm, stridor and convulsions. If the Q–T interval is prolonged, there may be ventricular arrhythmias. Further, chronically, it also causes basal ganglia calcification and cataracts. Acute, symptomatic hypocalcaemia is a medical emergency treated with intravenous calcium gluconate with electrocardiogram (ECG) monitoring, followed by intravenous infusion. Asymptomatic hypocalcaemia is treated with calcium and vitamin D, plus magnesium, if the magnesium level is low.

CHOLESTEROL/LIPIDS

The major lipids in the plasma are fatty acids, triglycerides, cholesterol and phospholipids. Elevated plasma levels of lipids, in particular cholesterol, are causally related to the development of atherosclerosis and thus coronary, cerebrovascular and peripheral vascular disease. Drug therapy aimed at reducing plasma cholesterol is contributing to the reduction in cardiovascular morbidity and mortality. The relationship between atherosclerotic disease and cholesterol may not extend into extreme old age: several epidemiological studies have found survival advantages in those with high cholesterol.

The metabolism and transport of lipids in the blood are complex and beyond the scope of this chapter. More details can be found in any larger medical textbook, as can details of the familial hyperlipidaemias.

Assessment

Blood sampling for lipid studies should be taken after an overnight fast, and alcohol should be avoided. Cholesterol levels fluctuate less in relation to food than to other plasma lipids. Strokes or myocardial infarctions can disturb lipid metabolism for up to 3 months, and sampling should take place within 24 hours of such an event or be deferred until then. Laboratory reports in the UK usually include low-density lipoprotein (LDL) cholesterol, high-density lipoprotein (HDL) cholesterol and triglyceride levels. HDL cholesterol is cardioprotective, and there is a lesser relationship between cardiovascular risk and triglycerides. Laboratories now provide a measure of the ratio between total cholesterol and HDL cholesterol (TC : HDL) to aid in determining cardiovascular risk.

Lipids are usually measured in patients with any atherosclerotic disease, where there is a family history of premature coronary artery disease (age < 60 years), where there are major risk factors for atherosclerotic disease, e.g. diabetes mellitus or hypertension, in patients with clinical features of hyperlipidaemia, e.g. tendon xanthomata, in those individuals in whom an incidental blood sample has been found to be lipaemic and to monitor the response to treatment of lipid-lowering agents.

Disorders of lipid metabolism may be primary (familial) or secondary. Obesity, alcohol excess, diabetes mellitus, hypothyroidism, cholestasis and chronic renal disease can lead to lipid abnormalities. Drugs such as thiazide diuretics and some beta-blockers can worsen hyperlipidaemia.

Management

The main aim of treating hyperlipidaemia is to reduce cardiovascular disease either through primary prevention before an event or secondary prevention after myocardial infarction, for example. Treatment is based on an overall assessment of risk and is not considered in isolation. Other vascular risk factors such as smoking, hypertension and diabetes mellitus should also be addressed. The benefit of cholesterol-lowering drugs, hydroxymethyl glutaryl coenzyme A (HMG-CoA) reductase inhibitors – statins, to achieve target reductions is well established in secondary prevention, and their prescription is now a routine matter. Details and current guidelines appear in the British National Formulary (BNF).

The cost benefit for primary prevention is much less, and in the UK, treatment is guided by coronary risk prediction. The BNF carries tables to guide treatment based on the 10-year risk. The value of primary prevention in elderly subjects has not been established. Other classes of drugs used include bile acid sequestrants such as cholestyramine, which reduces cholesterol but may increase triglyceride levels. Fibrates principally reduce triglycerides, with smaller effects on cholesterol. They do not have a clear effect on cardiovascular risk reduction and may be associated with an increased risk of non-cardiovascular deaths. Nicotinic acid reduces both cholesterol and triglycerides, but has not been assessed in outcome studies. Fish oils, the omega-3 fatty acids, reduce triglycerides.

HAEMOGLOBIN/ANAEMIA

In the presence of euvolaemia, anaemia is present in women if the haemoglobin level is below 120 g/l and in men if it is below 130 g/l. It is not a normal part of aging, and it should always be investigated and treated.

Symptoms and anaemia

The symptoms of anaemia depend on its severity:

(1)   Fatigue;

(2)   Difficulty concentrating;

(3)   Unusual food cravings;

(4)   Exertional breathlessness;

(5)   Weight loss;

(6)   Palpitations;

(7)   Angina;

(8)   Headache;

(9)   Dizziness;

(10) Syncope;

(11) Cognitive impairment.

You should ask whether the patient experiences any blood loss (haematemesis, melaena, rectal bleeding, haemoptysis, haematuria or postmenopausal bleeding) or has a condition associated with anaemia (alcohol excess, gastrointestinal (GI) surgery, liver disease, renal disease, chronic inflammatory disease or arthritis). You should also review medications for drugs associated with bleeding (e.g. non-steroidal anti-inflammatory drugs (NSAIDs)) or those that can suppress the bone marrow (e.g. anticonvulsants, major tranquillisers). (We cannot give a complete list of drugs associated with anaemia, so check each one that the patient is taking in the BNF.)

Examination of an anaemic patient

Examine the patient. Pallor is characteristic of anaemia but is not a reproducible sign. Further, many older people without anaemia appear pale (probably related to age-related endocrine changes). Pallor of the conjunctivae or buccal mucosa is a more reproducible sign: look for evidence of jaundice at the same time. Also look for clinical evidence of undernutrition. Features of acute blood loss include tachycardia, hypotension and postural hypotension. Feel for any enlarged lymph nodes. In chronic anaemia, the pulse may be bounding and there may be evidence of heart failure (high output). There is often a flow murmur audible at the base of the heart. Examine the abdomen for an enlarged liver or spleen and search for any other abdominal masses, and always perform a rectal examination (see page 56). If a female patient complains of vaginal bleeding or the nurses have noticed what appears to be vaginal bleeding, a pelvic examination will be required (best done by a gynaecologist).

Haematological indices

The report you receive after sending a sample for a full blood count (FBC) will contain much useful information. The mean corpuscular volume (MCV) will enable you to classify the anaemia into one of three groups:

(1) Microcytic (MCV < 80 fl);

(2) Macrocytic (MCV > 100 fl);

(3) Normocytic (MCV 80–100 fl).

If the mean corpuscular haemoglobin concentration (MCHC) is less than 30 g/dl, the anaemia is hypochromic.

The red cell distribution width is a measure of the variability of the size of the circulating red cells. Values above 14.5% suggest a dual population of cells, and are found in most types of anaemia that you are likely to encounter except the anaemia of chronic disease.

Microcytic anaemia

In your practice, the most likely cause is iron deficiency. It may also occur with copper deficiency, lead poisoning, sideroblastic anaemias and thalassaemia, although you should seek advice if any of these is a serious possibility. Otherwise, send blood for measurement of ferritin, which reflects iron stores: a level of < 10 µg/l diagnoses iron deficiency. Iron deficiency means blood loss until proved otherwise. Start oral iron supplements while searching for the site of blood loss. Only transfuse blood if the patient is symptomatic of anaemia.

Macrocytic anaemia

Macrocytic anaemia usually implies deficiency of vitamin B_{12} and/or folic acid. It can also arise in alcohol abuse, liver disease, hypothyroidism, hyperlipidaemia and myelodysplastic disorders. Send blood for the measurement of B_{12}, folate and red cell folate. Vitamin B_{12} deficiency may cause peripheral neuropathy, dorsal column degeneration in the spinal cord and dementia. If vitamin deficiency is found, treat following the guidance in the BNF. Also check for evidence of the other disorders listed, all of which necessitate treatment.

Normocytic anaemia

This arises in the early stages of microcytic and macrocytic anaemias, but more often reflects chronic disease (renal failure, liver failure, chronic inflammation, haemolysis) or acute blood loss. Acute blood loss should be readily apparent, and this should not be managed on a psychiatry ward: refer as appropriate. Other evidence should point towards haemolysis (page 38), liver disease (page 36) or renal disease (page 51), which, if present, necessitates an appropriate referral. The presence of a chronic inflammatory disorder will generally be indicated by an elevation of C-reactive protein (CRP).

LEUCOCYTOSIS

The white cells (leucocytes) present in the blood are produced in the bone marrow. The cells normally in the circulation are:

(1)   Neutrophils;

(2)   Lymphocytes;

(3)   Eosinophils;

(4)   Monocytes;

(5)   Basophils.

Most of the cells that normally circulate are neutrophils; lymphocytes are the second most populous cell type. About half of the circulating pool of neutrophils are loosely attached to vascular endothelium (marginated) and can be induced to detach themselves into the circulating blood on adrenergic stimulation. Glucocorticoids induce the release into the blood of immature neutrophils from the bone marrow.

Neutrophils are phagocytic cells involved in acute inflammation and have a short life. Monocytes are long-lived precursors of tissue macrophages which are also phagocytic; they are also crucial in the regulation of immune responses. Lymphocytes are the effector cells of immune responses.

The normal total white cell count (WBC) is $4.8–10.8 \times 10^9/l$. The normal neutrophil count is $4–6 \times 10^9/l$. The normal lymphocyte count is $2–5 \times 10^9/l$. A leucocytosis is a WBC that exceeds $10.8 \times 10^9/l$. Neutrophilia is present when their number exceeds $7.5 \times 10^9/l$. All of these counts are usually measured in autoanalysers.

Because each cell type can be increased in response to various stimuli, determining the predominant cell type in patients with a leucocytosis will point towards the likely cause. The commonest cell type to be elevated is the neutrophil. Common causes of a raised neutrophil count (neutrophilia) are:

(1)   Infections (bacteria, viruses, fungi, parasites);

(2)   Inflammation (gout, rheumatoid disease, vasculitis);

(3)   Drugs (glucocorticoids, lithium);

(4)   Metabolic (thyrotoxicosis, ketoacidosis);

(5)   Neoplasm (myeloproliferative disorder, myelodysplasia, renal cancer, GI cancer, lymphoma);

(6)   Haematological (haemolytic anaemia, splenectomy);

(7)   Trauma (tissue damage).

When assessing a patient with neutrophilia, think about infections first, unless something else is obviously the cause. Use the scheme we propose for searching for infections in fever of unknown origin (page 95). Only then should you consider the other causes listed above.

Lymphocytosis is less commonly encountered. Causes include:

(1)   Viral illness;

(2)   Tuberculosis (TB);

(3)   Toxoplasmosis;

(4)   Syphilis;

(5)   Chronic lymphocytic leukaemia;

(6)   Acute lymphocytic leukaemia;

(7)   Lymphoma;

(8)   Hepatitis.

If the cause is not apparent after considering these causes, a bone marrow investigation is indicated.

Monocytosis is not commonly encountered. Causes include:

(1)   TB;

(2)   Endocarditis;

(3)   Syphilis;

(4)   Fungal infection;

(5)   Protozoal infection;

(6)   Listeriosis;

(7)   Leukaemia;

(8)   Lymphoma;

(9)   Carcinoma;

(10) Sarcoidosis;

(11) Inflammatory bowel disease.

If the monocyte count is very high, think first of a haematological malignancy.

Eosinophilia is classically associated with parasitic diseases, but there are many other causes, which include:

(1)   Asthma;

(2)   Allergic rhinitis;

(3)   Atopic dermatitis;

(4)   Drug reactions;

(5)   Urticaria;

(6)   Bullous pemphigoid;

(7)   Scabies;

(8)   Helminthic infections (filariasis, ascariasis, schistosomiasis, strongy-
      loidiasis);

(9)   Lung disease (bronchopulmonary aspergillosis, eosinophilic pneumo-
      nia, Löffler's syndrome);

(10) Cholesterol embolism;

(11) Addison's disease;

(12) TB;

(13) Vasculitis;

(14) Rheumatoid disease;

(15) Eosinophilic fasciitis;

(16) Leukaemias;

(17) Lymphomas.

A full history and examination and other blood tests will often point to the
likely underlying explanation.

LIVER FUNCTION TESTS/JAUNDICE

The test battery used with most auto-analysers to indicate disorders of the
liver generally includes:

(1)   Albumin;

(2)   Bilirubin;

(3)   Alkaline phosphatase (AlkP);

(4)   Aspartate aminotransferase (AST);

(5)   Alanine aminotransferase (ALT);

(6)   Gamma-glutamyl transpeptidase (GGT).

None of them is a pure test of liver function.

Albumin

Albumin is manufactured in the liver and is the major protein found in the plasma. It has a long plasma half-life (about 20 days), so it is slow to react to liver injury or dysfunction. Albumin may be lost rapidly from the circulation because of capillary leaks (burns, gut inflammation) and kidney disease. The loss of more than 3 g per day in the urine defines nephrotic syndrome. If the albumin concentration falls sufficiently, because it contributes to plasma osmotic pressure, oedema results.

Bilirubin

Bilirubin is a product of haem (the oxygen-carrying part of haemoglobin) metabolism. Most is generated in the spleen as a result of erythrocyte degradation. It is insoluble in water and is transported to the liver bound to albumin, where it is conjugated to glucuronide (which is soluble in water) and secreted into the bile. In the colon, the glucuronide is removed by bacterial enzymes. It is then further metabolised to urobilinogen (some of which is reabsorbed) and urobilin. Bilirubin bound to albumin is not filtered by the renal glomeruli but conjugated bilirubin (glucuronide) is: its presence in urine reflects an increase in plasma conjugated bilirubin.

Increases in plasma bilirubin may arise in three circumstances:

(1)   Haemolysis;

(2)   Hepatic disease;

(3)   Biliary obstruction.

Jaundice, a yellow pigmentation, arises from the accumulation of bilirubin in body tissues. It is not usually clinically apparent before the bilirubin concentration in plasma exceeds 40 mmol/l. With haemolysis, the urine and faeces do not change colour. With liver damage, the urine may darken. With biliary obstruction, the faeces become pale and the urine darkens, and additionally, itching of the skin may be prominent.

Alkaline phosphatase

Alkaline phosphatase is found in many body tissues, but, in practice, elevations of alkaline phosphatase point to a disorder of either liver or bone. In liver disease, results of other items of the test battery listed above are very likely to be abnormal. With biliary obstruction, the alkaline phosphatase result is likely to be greater than three times the upper limit of normal, whereas with hepatocellular disease, it is usually less than three times the upper limit of normal.

Transaminases

AST and ALT are the main transaminases measured routinely. AST is present in the mitochondria and cytosol of hepatocytes and other cells (skeletal muscle, heart and pancreas), whereas ALT is present only in the cytosol, mainly of hepatocytes. Transaminases do not rise with haemolysis.

In hepatitis, the ALT concentration is generally greater than that of AST. The reverse situation occurs with widespread hepatocellular necrosis. Further, with hepatocellular disease, transaminases generally rise 10–100 times the upper limit of normal, whereas in biliary obstruction, they generally do not rise to greater than ten-fold the upper limit of normal.

Gamma-glutamyl transpeptidase

This enzyme is found in many body tissues, but elevations in plasma levels only occur with liver disease or as a result of enzyme induction by drugs or alcohol. Thus, in the case of an elevated alkaline phosphatase level, a normal GGT strongly suggests a bony origin.

Clinical features

Haemolysis

Acute haemolysis is rare, and, in the setting of an old age psychiatry service, it is only likely to arise following transfusion of mismatched blood. The features of this are: hypotension, back pain, chest pain, oliguria and haemoglobinuria. If this situation is suspected, the transfusion must be stopped immediately. The blood should be returned to the blood bank and samples of venous blood must be taken for full blood count and coagulation studies. In addition, an anticoagulant-free blood sample should also be sent in a plain tube. A haematologist, who will decide about further management, must be contacted as a matter of urgency as the situation is potentially life-threatening, although not inevitably so, and very old people have recovered from it.

More likely, although still uncommon, is subacute and chronic haemolysis, usually referred to as haemolytic anaemia. In this condition, the lifespan of erythrocytes is considerably shortened. Although the bone marrow can increase red cell production about seven-fold, it is usually an inadequate response and anaemia results. The high turnover of red cells also increases the demand for folic acid, which, if unmet, results in folate deficiency and its consequences. The laboratory findings include an increase in bilirubin (unconjugated) and lactate dehydrogenase (LDH) as a result of erythrocyte degradation. Plasma haptoglobins are low or absent as they bind haemoglobin avidly. The blood film will show polychromasia and the reticulocyte count will be increased. Most patients will be clinically anaemic and the spleen will be enlarged (except in sickle cell disease). The haemolytic anaemias are clearly outside the competence of an old age psychiatry service and the patient should be referred to a haematologist for further diagnosis and treatment.

Hepatocellular disease

In an old age psychiatry service, medications and alcohol are the most likely causes of acute liver disease, although acute infective hepatitis may also be seen. The likely cause is usually apparent, often after the introduction of a new drug. The list of possible drugs that may cause acute hepatocellular damage is very long and you should check them in the BNF. You should stop all potentially harmful drugs and repeat the liver function tests after a few days if the patient is clinically well. If the patient is unwell, medical advice must be sought. Sometimes, the situation can progress very rapidly, resulting in fulminant liver failure, even without jaundice being clinically apparent. Any patient with evidence of hepatocellular damage and features of an encephalopathy must be seen very urgently by a gastroenterologist. He will find it useful to know the results of the following investigations: bilirubin, transaminases, alkaline phosphatase, prothrombin time, electrolytes and blood glucose. Blood gases, if available, would also be appreciated.

A situation that an old age psychiatrist will more often encounter is a patient who is already known to have chronic liver disease who suddenly deteriorates. Again, medications are most likely to be the underlying cause, but infection, gastrointestinal bleeding or electrolyte disturbances could also explain the deterioration. In this situation, you need an urgent referral to a gastroenterologist. Try to have the results of the investigations listed in the previous paragraph. You should never start new drugs for a patient known to have chronic liver disease without consulting Appendix 2 of the BNF.

Biliary obstruction

This is usually caused by mechanical obstruction of the biliary tract outside the liver. Intrahepatic cholestasis is rare, and is most often caused by drugs. Benign obstruction outside the liver most often occurs as a result of a gallstone migrating into the common bile duct. When associated with fever and chills, it is known as cholangitis. Classically, a carcinoma of the head of the pancreas or of the ampulla of Vater can cause mechanical obstruction of the biliary tree. If the gall bladder is palpable, it suggests that the cause is not gallstones and makes malignant obstruction more likely (Courvoisier's law), but you must not rely on this being so. The initial approach to both types of obstruction is via an endoscope, so referral to a gastroenterologist is necessary.

PLATELETS

Platelets are formed by budding from the surface of megakaryocytes in the bone marrow. They play a critical role in blood coagulation. Thrombocytopenia is defined by a platelet count below $150\,000/\mu l$. The clinical features of thrombocytopaenia depend on how low the platelet count is. Counts above $50\,000/\mu l$ are not usually associated with symptoms. Counts between $20\,000$ and $50\,000/\mu l$ are associated with easy bruising, but not usually with overt bleeding. Counts below $20\,000/\mu l$ are often associated with overt bleeding. The platelet count may fall because of decreased production, sequestration in the spleen (hypersplenism of any cause) and increased destruction.

Causes of reduced platelet production include:

(1) Aplastic anaemia (red cell count and WBC also low);

(2) Neoplasms (leukaemia, myelodysplasia, metastatic cancer);

(3) Vitamin deficiency (B_{12}, folate);

(4) Drugs (check in BNF);

(5) Severe infections.

Causes of increased platelet destruction include:

(1)   Microangiopathic haemolytic anaemia (disseminated intravascular coagulation, haemolytic–uraemic syndrome);

(2)   Immune destruction (rheumatoid disease, medications, idiopathic thrombocytopenic purpura, heparin).

Patients with thrombocytopenia require a detailed physical examination, paying special attention to the spleen and lymph nodes. If the cause is not readily apparent, get a haematology opinion, urgently if there is bleeding, if the patient is very ill or if the platelet count is 20 000/μl or less.

POTASSIUM

Potassium is the major intracellular cation, and it is critical for normal neuromuscular function. It is very difficult to have a dietary excess or deficit of potassium sufficient to cause symptoms. Because of exchanges of potassium with protons across cell membranes, there is generally an inverse relationship between potassium and bicarbonate in the blood plasma. More than 90% of the potassium filtered by the glomeruli is reabsorbed in the proximal nephron. The potassium content of urine is regulated hormonally in the distal nephron: aldosterone promotes potassium losses in the urine. Further, insulin promotes potassium uptake by many cell types, but mainly skeletal muscle.

Hyperkalaemia

Hyperkalaemia is present with a plasma potassium concentration > 5.5 mmol/l and arises in four main situations:
(1)   Spurious:

(a)   Haemolysis during venesection;

(b)   Leakage from red cells;

(2)   Decreased excretion:

(a)   Renal failure;

(b)   Secretory defects (interstitial nephritis);

(c)   Hypoaldosteronism (renal tubular acidosis, diabetic nephropathy, Addison's disease);

    (d)   Drugs (spironolactone, triamterene, amiloride, angiotensin-converting enzyme inhibitors (ACEIs), trimethoprim, NSAIDs);

(3)   Shift from cells:

    (a)   Burns (rhabdomyolysis);

    (b)   Metabolic acidosis;

    (c)   Digoxin;

(4)   Excess intake:

    (a)   Potassium supplements;

    (b)   Potassium added to intravenous infusions.

You will usually encounter hyperkalaemia as a biochemical disorder rather than recognising the clinical features and doing the blood test. The clinical features of hyperkalaemia are weakness, possibly flaccid paralysis, abdominal distension and diarrhoea. The ECG may be normal, but more often shows peaked T waves and sometimes wide QRS complexes and bradycardia. There is a risk of developing lethal ventricular fibrillation and cardiac arrest.

The cause will usually be recognised from the circumstances. Look at the urea and creatinine concentrations: if elevated, suspect renal failure or Addison's disease. If a patient is taking ACEIs, spironolactone, triamterene or amiloride, they are likely to be the precipitating cause, but there is often underlying renal impairment. You will be aware if you are giving potassium supplements.

If the plasma potassium is < 6.0 mmol/l, the situation is not urgent. You need to restrict potassium intake and withdraw potassium-retaining drugs. As the potassium-retaining drugs were given for a reason, withdrawing them might cause a new problem: get medical advice.

If the plasma potassium is > 6.5 mmol/l, you have a medical emergency on your hands, and the patient must be transferred to medical care as soon as possible. The myocardium can be stabilised by giving 10 ml of 10% calcium gluconate intravenously. Plasma potassium can be lowered by giving 50 ml of 50% glucose with 10 u of short-acting insulin. Calcium resonium is given by mouth (15 g 3–4 times daily) or rectum. Dialysis may be needed. Plasma potassium measurements between 6.0 and 6.5 mmol/l are serious but less urgent: seek medical advice quickly.

Hypokalaemia

This is present if the plasma potassium is < 3.5 mmol/l. It arises in four settings:

(1) Inadequate intake:

  (a) Undernutrition;

  (b) Eating disorders;

(2) Renal losses:

  (a) Diuretics;

  (b) Mineralocorticoid excess (Conn's syndrome, Cushing's syndrome, ectopic adrenocorticotropic hormone (ACTH) production, renal artery stenosis, hypertension, heart failure);

  (c) Renal tubular acidosis;

(3) Gastrointestinal losses:

  (a) Diarrhoea;

  (b) Vomiting;

  (c) Laxative abuse;

  (d) Villous adenoma;

(4) Redistribution:

  (a) Insulin treatment;

  (b) Acute illness;

  (c) β_2 Adrenoreceptor agonists.

The commonest cause is diuretic use, and this is the first thing to look for. If this is not the case, gastrointestinal causes other than laxative abuse will usually be obvious. Those who are undernourished or have eating disorders will show signs of undernutrition. The renal disorders can be rather more difficult to diagnose. Request a measurement of urine potassium: if the loss of potassium is not through the kidneys, urine potassium should be very low. You will need medical help to investigate things further, and a simultaneous measurement of urine and plasma potassium and osmolality should be requested: it helps in calculation of the transtubular potassium concentration gradient (TTKG), which may assist diagnosis.

Hypokalaemia is often asymptomatic, even when severe. The commonest features are weakness, constipation and intestinal ileus. The ECG may show T wave flattening and U waves. Long-standing hypokalaemia can damage the distal nephron, leading to an impairment of the urine-concentrating mechanism, polyuria and polydipsia. If the plasma potassium concentration is severely low (< 2.0 mmol/l), profound muscle weakness, flaccid paralysis and respiratory failure may arise.

If the plasma potassium concentration is between 2.5 and 3.5 mmol/l, give oral potassium supplements (80–120 mmol/day in divided doses). If the plasma potassium is below 2.5 mmol/l, intravenous treatment is indicated (no more than 20 mmol/hour at a concentration of no more than 40 mmol/l). You may choose to seek advice if the plasma potassium concentration is below 3.0 mmol/l. The underlying cause of the hypokalaemia needs to be elucidated and corrected, where possible.

SODIUM AND WATER

Sodium is the major extracellular cation: 80–90% is located in the extracellular compartment. There does not seem to be a control mechanism that regulates sodium intake. Thus, to maintain a constant body sodium content, intake must be balanced by output. Small amounts of sodium are lost in sweat and faeces, but the major excretory route is via the kidney. About 70% of filtered sodium is reabsorbed in the proximal convoluted tubule. Because of concurrent water absorption, the tubular fluid remains iso-osmotic with the plasma. Some 20–30% of the filtered sodium is reabsorbed in the loop of Henlé. This sodium is trapped in the renal interstitium and, along with urea, contributes to the medullary osmotic gradient, which is needed for concentration of the urine. In addition, 5–10% of the filtered sodium is reabsorbed in the distal convoluted tubule, which also secretes potassium into the tubular fluid. The reabsorption of sodium and loss of potassium is modulated by the adrenal cortical hormone, aldosterone. Aldosterone also regulates sodium absorption in the collecting ducts. Atrial natriuretic peptides and brain natriuretic peptides also regulate sodium reabsorption/loss. Thus, the major factors regulating renal sodium handling are:

(1) Glomerular filtration rate;

(2) Aldosterone;

(3) Natriuretic peptides.

Sodium metabolism is intricately bound up with that of water. Water metabolism is determined mainly by sensing the osmolality of the plasma (hypothalamic osmoreceptors) and the blood volume (blood pressure). The normal plasma osmolality is about 285 ± 10 mOsm/kg. The urinary osmolality depends on the state of hydration (50–1200 mOsm/kg). The main hormone regulating water metabolism is antidiuretic hormone (vasopressin), which is secreted by the posterior pituitary gland in response to increased osmolality and reduced blood pressure. Clinical disorders of body sodium always involve water metabolism.

Aging is associated with reduced renal blood flow, reduced abilities to concentrate and dilute the urine and an impaired ability to secrete an acid load.

Hypernatraemia

This is present when the plasma sodium is > 145 mmol/l. It occurs in three circumstances:

(1) Hypovolaemia (sodium and water deficit):

    (a) Diuretics;

    (b) Osmotic diuresis;

    (c) Post-urinary obstruction;

    (d) Sweating;

    (e) Burns;

    (f) Diarrhoea;

    (g) Fistulae;

(2) Euvolaemia (water deficit):

    (a) Diabetes insipidus;

    (b) Nephrogenic diabetes insipidus;

    (c) Impaired thirst;

    (d) Evaporation from skin and lungs;

(3) Hypervolaemia (sodium excess):

    (a) Excessive NaCl infusion:

    (b) Hypertonic dialysis;

    (c)   Cushing's syndrome;

    (d)   Hyperaldosteronism.

Hypernatraemia seldom develops unless thirst is impaired or access to water is restricted. This electrolyte abnormality is associated with a high risk of death, and is best managed by physicians, not psychiatrists. You should make an urgent referral to arrange this.

In geriatric practice, hypernatraemia is most often encountered in those unable to replace water losses, often with an acute illness in residential or nursing-home care. It is also a prominent feature of hyperosmolar, non-ketotic diabetic coma (HONK), which is discussed in more detail on page 84. Apart from hypernatraemia arising in the context of diuretic use, the other causes are relatively uncommon.

If there is an expanded plasma volume, the excess sodium is usually eliminated by using diuretics. If the patient is euvolaemic, 5% dextrose is given to reduce the circulating plasma sodium by no more than 0.5 mmol/h. If there is hypovolaemia and/or the plasma sodium is above 170 mmol/l, it is corrected with 0.9% saline. Thereafter, water or salt-free solutions are provided.

Hyponatraemia

This is present when the plasma sodium is < 130 mmol/l. It arises in three circumstances:

(1)   Hypovolaemia (sodium and water deficit):

    (a)   Vomiting;

    (b)   Diarrhoea;

    (c)   Dehydration + sweating;

    (d)   Osmotic diuresis;

    (e)   Diuretics;

    (f)   Tubulointerstitial renal disease;

    (g)   Cerebral salt-wasting syndrome;

    (h)   Addison's disease;

(2)   Euvolaemia (modest water excess):

    (a)   Syndrome of inappropriate antidiuresis (SIA);

(b) Antidepressants;

(c) Anticonvulsants;

(d) Abnormal antidiuretic hormone (ADH) release (vagal neuropathy, hypothyroidism, severe potassium deficiency, Addison's disease, hyperglycaemia, alcohol, sick cell syndrome);

(3) Hypervolaemia (water and sodium excess):

(a) Heart failure;

(b) Liver failure;

(c) Oliguric renal failure;

(d) Hypoalbuminaemia.

Hyponatraemia is often asymptomatic, and discovered as an incidental blood test abnormality. The clinical features depend on the underlying mechanism, and it is conventional to assign patients to one of three groups according to their 'volume' status: hypovolaemia, euvolaemia and hypervolaemia. Further elucidation of the likely cause is aided by measuring the urine sodium concentration. We recommend that you seek a medical opinion on all hyponatraemic patients, as diagnosis and treatment can be difficult and challenging. The more severe the hyponatraemia or the symptoms associated with it, the more is the urgency of your need for advice.

The features of hypovolaemia are thirst, raised heart rate, hypotension, postural hypotension, reduced skin turgor and reduced jugular venous pressure. If the urine sodium concentration exceeds 20 mmol/l, likely causes include diuretics, salt-losing nephritis, cerebral salt-wasting syndrome and Addison's disease (refer for advice). Urine sodium concentrations less than 20 mmol/l are associated with sweating, vomiting and diarrhoea. This situation is treated with intravenous sodium chloride and correction of the underlying cause.

In the presence of hypervolaemia there is oedema, hypertension and elevated jugular venous pressure. If the urine sodium concentration exceeds 20 mmol/l, renal failure is likely to explain the situation. Urine sodium less than 20 mmol/l is associated with heart failure, liver failure, nephrotic syndrome and incompetent intravenous fluid administration. The treatment here is generally with diuretics and fluid restriction: this is better done on a medical ward.

Euvolaemic hyponatraemia is treated with fluid restriction as well as the treatment of any underlying disorder. Sometimes, demeclocycline or lithium is also given. The syndrome of inappropriate antidiuresis (SIA) is often misdiagnosed. It requires inappropriately concentrated urine (> 100 mOsm/kg) for the hypo-osmolar plasma (< 270 mOsm/kg). In addition, the urine sodium is > 20 mmol/l and there must be no evidence of thyroid, pituitary or adrenal disease. The patient should not be taking diuretics.

Hyponatraemia, when it develops slowly, is often markedly asymptomatic. Treatment with sodium chloride will be determined by the severity of the hyponatraemia and the presence of symptoms of hyponatraemia. Generally, sodium treatment is not needed with plasma sodium concentrations > 125 mmol/l, and sometimes lower depending on the cause and the symptoms. The presence of confusion, ataxia, weakness and muscle cramps suggest that treatment should be given: such symptoms occur with sodium concentrations between 110 and 125 mmol/l. Sodium concentrations below 110 mmol/l are more likely to be associated with coma, convulsions and death. A serious complication of hyponatraemia (and its too-rapid correction) is central pontine myelinolysis, characterised by quadriplegia, cranial nerve palsies and sometimes other encephalopathic features. The plasma sodium should not increase faster than 0.5 mmol/hour if the hyponatraemia is chronic, although more rapid correction rates are appropriate if the hyponatraemia developed rapidly.

THYROID

The thyroid gland lies in the anterior neck and overlies the trachea. It takes the approximate shape of the letter H. It is responsible for the synthesis and secretion of thyroid hormones, under the control of the anterior pituitary gland and hypothalamus. In addition, parafollicular cells secrete calcitonin in response to changes in ionised calcium concentration. Thyrotrophin-releasing hormone (TRH) from the hypothalamus induces the synthesis and secretion into the blood of the glycoprotein called thyrotrophin (thyroid-stimulating hormone, TSH). TRH may have direct effects on parts of the brain, and it has been suggested as a mediator of Hashimoto's encephalopathy. TSH binds to receptors in the membrane of thyroid follicular cells and stimulates the synthesis and secretion of thyroid hormones. There is inhibitory feedback by thyroid hormones at the level of the pituitary and, probably, the hypothalamus too.

Thyroid hormones are formed by the coupling of monoiodotyrosine and di-iodotyrosine to form T_3 and T_4 (tri-iodothyronine and thyroxine). This coupling is inhibited by propylthiouracil and carbimazole, drugs used to treat hyperthyroidism. Nearly all of the circulating thyroid hormones are bound to plasma proteins, mainly thyroid-binding globulin (TBG). It is only the unbound hormone that is metabolically active.

Thyroid hormones are metabolised in the tissues. T_3 is formed from T_4 by β-deiodination and it is highly active. α-Deiodination forms reverse T_3 (rT_3), which is inactive. Many forms of illness influence the peripheral metabolism of thyroid hormones, which can make the interpretation of thyroid function tests difficult. We recommend that you do not perform thyroid function tests in ill patients unless you think that the illness is caused by thyroid disease. A further difficulty is that many drugs affect the secretion and metabolism of thyroid hormones.

Thyroid disease is hard to diagnose in older people, as many of the features are common among those without thyroid disease; some thyrotoxic patients present clinically as myxoedema (apathetic thyrotoxicosis). Hence, screening tests are well worthwhile. Symptoms associated with thyroid disease include weakness, fatigue, depression/irritability, cold/heat intolerance, dry skin/sweating, hair loss, constipation/diarrhoea and weight gain/loss. The thyroid gland is usually not palpably enlarged.

Hypothyroidism

Many laboratories measure TSH to screen for hypothyroidism, and a level > 5 mU/l usually indicates hypothyroidism. If the T_3 and T_4 measurements are normal, this is generally referred to as subclinical hypothyroidism. Over time, many such patients progress to overt hypothyroidism, especially those with high titres of antithyroid antibodies. Many authors recommend treating these patients with thyroxine, while others pursue a policy of watch and wait.

Hypothyroidism is clearly present when the TSH is raised and the levels of thyroid hormones are reduced. Further investigation is generally not needed, as most cases turn out to be autoimmune thyroid failure (Hashimoto's disease). Treatment is usually started with 50 μg of L-thyroxine. Dose increases of 25 μg should occur every 4–6 weeks, guided by the TSH level. Once the patient is stable, TSH can be checked every 6 months.

Myxoedema coma is an extreme form of hypothyroidism, fortunately very rare, that may sometimes develop very rapidly, often after severe illness, infection, trauma or surgery. It is a life-threatening decompensated state that must be diagnosed clinically. The reason for mentioning it here is that it is an easily overlooked diagnosis which is eminently treatable.

Because of the seriousness of the situation, you need to request the help of the on-call physicians if you suspect this diagnosis.

The typical patient is a woman who becomes confused, obtunded or frankly comatose, often after an infection, accident, injury or some other severe illness. There may coexist signs that can be attributed to heart failure or respiratory failure. If myxoedema coma is suspected, blood needs to be sent for TSH, T_3 and T_4 measurement. As these results will not be available for some days, other results can help in supporting the diagnosis. In myxoedema coma, there is usually hyponatraemia, hypothermia, raised creatine kinase, hypoglycaemia, hypercholesterolaemia and mild anaemia (normocytic/macrocytic). Blood gases show reduced oxygen partial pressure (pO_2) and raised carbon dioxide partial pressure (pCO_2). The ECG shows bradycardia, often with a prolonged Q-T interval. The chest radiograph may show pleural or pericardial effusions.

Treatment is with intravenous thyroxine (200–400 µg) under ECG monitoring, followed by 100 µg daily intravenously. Supportive care is undertaken, and any associated conditions are treated.

Hyperthyroidism

This diagnosis is suggested by a low TSH (< 0.1 mU/l). If the levels of T_3 and T_4 are normal, this is referred to as subclinical hyperthyroidism. There is no consensus on how this should be managed, and you should seek advice. When the levels of thyroid hormones are elevated, hyperthyroidism (thyrotoxicosis) is present. Occasionally, T_4 is normal or low and the T_3 is raised (T_3 toxicosis). Unlike in the young, the most likely cause of thyrotoxicosis in older people is not Grave's disease, but toxic multinodular goitre. Multinodular goitres are common among older people, but thyrotoxicosis is not always associated with them.

Treatment is best done by a physician. β-Adrenergic antagonists ameliorate tremor, palpitations and agitation: thyroid hormones sensitise adrenergic receptors to their natural agonists. Treatment with carbimazole or propylthiouracil is usually then started and the T_4 starts to fall in 2–4 weeks. The dose is reduced once the patient is euthyroid. These antithyroid drugs cause rashes, fever and arthralgias in about 5% of older people treated with them. Occasionally, agranulocytosis occurs, so the white blood cell count needs regular monitoring.

Long-term treatment with antithyroid drugs is not usually done. More often, patients are referred for radioactive iodine ablation of the thyroid or, sometimes, surgery. The antithyroid drugs need to be stopped 3–5 days before radioactive iodine administration.

Hashimoto's encephalopathy

Hashimoto's encephalopathy was first described in 1966 and it is rare, although probably underdiagnosed because people are unaware of it. Cognitive impairment is a frequently reported feature. There seem to be two different clinical presentations. The 'vasculitic' type is characterised by relapsing–remitting stroke-like episodes. The diffuse-progressive type shows insidious or fluctuating cognitive impairment, confusion, psychosis, somnolence and sometimes coma. Rarely, epileptic seizures occur, and the disorder has been recorded as presenting with status epilepticus.

Patients may be euthyroid, but they have very high titres of antimicrosomal antibodies and antibodies to thyroglobulin. Most patients with Hashimoto's encephalopathy have normal magnetic resonance imaging (MRI) scans and computed tomography (CT) scans. The cerebrospinal fluid is abnormal in most patients: the protein level is high and there is a mononuclear cell pleocytosis. The electroencephalogram (EEG) is usually abnormal, and reflects the degree of central nervous system (CNS) involvement. The EEG findings include mild to severe generalised slowing, triphasic waves and epileptiform abnormalities. The pathogenesis of Hashimoto's encephalopathy is unknown.

Usually, patients with Hashimoto's encephalopathy respond to glucocorticoids (initially in high doses); however, various immunosuppressive treatments have been used, including azathioprine, cyclophosphamide, intravenous immunoglobulin and plasmapheresis.

UREA/CREATININE/RENAL DISEASE

Urea is an end product of nitrogen metabolism, which is produced in the liver and excreted in the kidneys. Creatinine is formed mainly in skeletal muscle by the non-enzymatic hydrolysis of creatine; it is also excreted in the kidneys. Creatinine concentration reflects not only the ability of the kidneys to excrete it, but also the body mass of skeletal muscle (lean body mass), which declines during aging. Therefore, creatinine concentration may not rise predictably until renal failure is severe. In recognition of this, some laboratories have started to report an estimated glomerular filtration rate based on the creatinine concentration and other information you are expected to supply on the laboratory request form: make sure you fill in such forms properly.

Clinically, urea and creatinine are used as markers of kidney function; and the term uraemia implies an elevation in the urea concentration, and is a virtual proxy for the term renal failure. It is not an exact proxy because the urea concentration can rise after a large protein-rich meal or a gastrointestinal haemorrhage (which can also cause renal failure by reducing kidney perfusion).

The kidneys can fail for three main reasons:

(1)   Reduced perfusion (pre-renal);

(2)   Intrinsic renal disease (renal);

(3)   Obstruction to urine drainage (post-renal; obstructive uropathy).

Acute renal failure

All patients will be best managed by a physician than by a psychiatrist, and should be referred promptly. It will be appreciated that you will have not only the results of urea, creatinine and electrolyte measurements, but also the results of a full blood count and urine stick testing. The early symptoms in acute renal failure usually reflect the underlying cause: symptoms of the renal failure develop later and include nausea, vomiting and delirium. Bleeding can arise because of altered platelet function. Hyperkalaemia usually develops with significant renal impairment (page 41). Acidosis, which occurs because the metabolic acid load cannot be excreted adequately, causes tachypnoea. Urine output falls in hypotensive or infective causes ($< 500\,ml$ per 24 hours defines oliguria). With other forms of acute renal failure, oliguria is less common. Myoclonic jerks are commonly observed. Uraemic encephalopathy has a very poor prognosis: the earliest sign is asterixis.

Characteristically in acute renal failure, the urea and creatinine concentrations progressively rise. If the cause is pre-renal or post-renal, the urea concentration increases disproportionately to that of creatinine and the urea/creatinine ratio will be $> 20 : 1$. On stick testing of the urine, if there is a significant amount of protein, glomerulonephritis is a likely cause, although cholesterol embolism syndrome may present similarly (eosinophilia is a clue to this). If pre-renal uraemia is not promptly treated, acute renal tubular necrosis develops and dirty-brown granular casts appear as urinary sediment.

The underlying cause of pre-renal uraemia will often be apparent: the kidneys are inadequately perfused because of reduced circulating blood volume (haemorrhage, dehydration, diuretics) or reduced cardiac output (heart failure).

Acute tubular necrosis occurs by progression of pre-renal uraemia, or following the use of nephrotoxic drugs (aminoglycosides, NSAIDs, ACEIs). With acute glomerulonephritis, the presentation will be with nephritic syndrome or nephrotic syndrome. The nephritic syndrome presents abruptly with hypertension, haematuria, uraemia and fluid retention (oedema). Nephrotic syndrome has a more gradual onset with increasing oedema, albuminuria (> 3 g/day) and hypoalbuminaemia. All patients with glomerulonephritis need a renal biopsy and management by a nephrologist.

In a case of obstructive uropathy, the abdomen should always be examined for an enlarged bladder and other abdominal masses; a rectal examination should be done to assess the prostate and to detect any malignant disease in the pelvis. Oliguria or anuria is common, although some patients have a normal or increased urine output (increased tubular pressure from obstruction can cause tubular dysfunction and nephrogenic diabetes insipidus). If obstructive uropathy is considered possible, a urinary catheter needs to be passed to relieve bladder outlet obstruction followed by careful fluid balance. A renal ultrasound will detect hydronephrosis. You will need medical/surgical input to manage these patients.

Chronic renal failure

Most patients with chronic renal failure are elderly and the most common underlying cause is diabetes mellitus. Fatigue and weakness are the commonest symptoms. With progression, nausea, vomiting and itching emerge as prominent symptoms. Urinary frequency and nocturia are common because of impaired urinary concentrating ability (isosthenuria). When very advanced, irritability, drowsiness and coma may ensue. Without treatment, seizures may also emerge.

On examination, patients have a sallow complexion, bruising and evidence of scratching the skin. Hypertension is usually present. The patients are usually anaemic. The patients have impaired vitamin D metabolism and develop secondary hyperparathyroidism and osteomalacia. Calcium may be deposited in small arteries in the skin leading to extremely painful skin necrosis (calciphylaxis; treated by parathyroidectomy). Inadequate production of erythropoietin results in anaemia. Hyperkalaemia is unusual until very late in the disorder.

For most of the patients you see, the diagnosis will have been made already and the patient will already be under the care of a nephrologist or a geriatrician. They may well be taking phosphate-binding drugs and 1α-hydroxyvitamin D (to prevent osteodystrophy), sodium bicarbonate (to treat acidosis), DDAVP (desmopressin, for bruising), antihypertensives and erythropoietin (to treat anaemia). If you make a new presumptive diagnosis of chronic renal failure, you must refer the patient. It will be appreciated if you have the results of measurements of urea, creatinine, electrolytes, calcium and phosphate as well as the results of urine stick testing and a full blood count.

4   Clinical management

BENIGN PROSTATIC HYPERTROPHY

Prostatic enlargement occurs inevitably with advancing age, and becomes
progressively symptomatic. About 50% of men aged 50–60 years and 80%
of octogenarians have complaints referable to the prostate gland. The
symptoms produced may be both irritative and filling:

(1)   Incomplete emptying;

(2)   Intermittent urinary stream (stop and start again);

(3)   Frequency;

(4)   Urgency;

(5)   Poor stream;

(6)   Straining;

(7)   Post-micturition dribbling;

(8)   Urinary retention.

Many of these symptoms can have other causes such as bladder stone, bladder cancer and prostate cancer, so the initial assessment focuses on estab-
lishing that the symptoms are not due to these other causes.

    Patient examination should include an abdominal examination to pal-
pate the bladder and a rectal examination to assess prostate size, shape and
consistency. In benign hypertrophy, the gland is symmetrically enlarged,
smooth and rubbery in consistency. A tender, firm prostate most likely indicates prostatitis, and a hard, nodular gland suggests cancer. Urinalysis
should be performed to detect haematuria which will require further investigation, and to find evidence of infection. Urea and electrolytes should be
checked. Prostate-specific antigen (PSA) can be measured, especially if rectal examination suggests a malignant prostate.

    No treatment may be required for mild symptoms, which may not
progress. Further options depend on the patient's fitness for surgery.

Medical treatment with α-adrenoreceptor blocking drugs (which produce side-effects in up to 20% of patients) and/or 5α-reductase inhibitors (finasteride) may improve symptoms, sometimes dramatically. α1-Receptors are present in the smooth muscle of the prostatic stroma and capsule as well as in the urethra and bladder neck; noradrenaline stimulation causes these muscles to contract, obstructing the bladder outlet. Finasteride blocks the conversion of testosterone to the more potent androgen, dihydrotestosterone. Treatment combining both drugs produces a higher response rate and better symptom control than treatment with either class of drug alone. Transurethral resection of the prostate is the usual surgical treatment, although open prostatectomy is sometimes done for very large glands. Some patients, especially those developing urinary retention and who are not fit for surgery, may be treated with a long-term, indwelling urinary catheter.

How to do a rectal examination

The commonest position for digital examination of the rectum is the left lateral (Sims') position. The patient lies on the left side with the right upper leg flexed, and the left (lower) leg is semi-extended. This allows a detailed examination of the anus as well as of the rectum. A gloved and lubricated index finger is passed into the rectum. The rectum can also be examined in the modified lithotomy position with the patient lying supine with flexed knees; it is difficult to perform a detailed examination of the anus in this position. The examiner's right hand is passed under the patient's right thigh and a gloved and lubricated index finger is passed into the rectum. Finally, the patient can be examined standing bending over the bed/examination couch.

The anal skin should be examined for evidence of inflammation and other rashes (e.g. lichen sclerosus et atrophicus, Paget's disease of skin), excoriation, fissures, nodules, fistulae, scars, tumours, rectal prolapse and haemorrhoids. Ask the patient to strain (bear down) while you inspect for haemorrhoids and fissures. Any abnormal areas should be palpated. Then tell the patient you are about to examine the inside of the rectum (using whatever euphemisms are acceptable). The patient should also be told about the cold sensation of the lubricant followed shortly by the sensation of having to move the bowels: reassure the person that the bowels will not actually move. The left hand is used to separate the buttocks and the right index finger is placed on the anal verge; gentle pressure tends to relax the anal sphincter. Ask the patient to take a deep breath, during which the finger is inserted. The sphincter should close around the examining finger.

Assess sphincter tone and then ask the patient to squeeze the finger to assess sphincter strength. Note the amount and consistency of any faeces present. Examine systematically the posterior lateral and anterior walls. The ischial spines, coccyx and lower sacrum can be easily felt through the rectal wall. Feel for masses, irregularities and undue tenderness. Because of the limitations on your wrist movements, the area between 12 o'clock and 3 o'clock is difficult to examine. Sometimes, intraperitoneal metastases can be felt in the pouch of Douglas.

The prostate can be felt through the anterior wall. Note its size, shape, surface, consistency and sensitivity. The normal prostate is smooth, rubbery and heart-shaped (the apex of the heart points to the anus). The seminal vesicles lie above the prostate and cannot normally be felt.

Finally, inform the patient when you will withdraw the finger. Having withdrawn it, inspect the finger for the colour of any faecal matter and look for blood.

BREATHLESSNESS – ACUTE

Acute breathlessness must always be taken very seriously, as many of the causes are potentially lethal. A psychiatry ward is not an appropriate environment to manage these patients. The causes include:

(1) Respiratory (pneumothorax, pulmonary embolism, bronchospasm, aspiration, pneumonia, upper airway obstruction);

(2) Cardiac (myocardial infarction, heart failure, dysrhythmia, pericardial tamponade);

(3) Metabolic (acidosis);

(4) Infective (septicaemia, pneumonia);

(5) Anaemia;

(6) Anxiety (hyperventilation).

Evaluating an acutely breathless patient

The details of the onset of the breathlessness must be noted. Is the patient febrile or suffering from chest pain? Is there cyanosis? Is there purulent sputum (infection) or haemoptysis (pulmonary embolus, cancer, heart failure)? Is the heart rate very rapid? Is there any wheezing or stridor? Is the level of consciousness impaired? Check oxygen saturation if you have access to a pulse oximeter.

Markedly abnormal vital signs (temperature, pulse, blood pressure) are ominous features in a very breathless patient, indicating the urgency with which the patient needs to be transferred to the acute medical service or accident and emergency (A&E) department. Listen to the lung fields for crackles or wheezes. Wheezing usually indicates asthma, but is common in patients with chronic obstructive pulmonary disease (COPD). Diminished breath sounds on only one side of the chest suggest pneumothorax, a large pleural effusion or lung collapse. In heart failure, pulmonary embolus and pericardial tamponade, the jugular venous pressure will often be obviously raised.

Treating the acutely breathless patient

Insert an intravenous (iv) cannula to ensure venous access in case the patient deteriorates. If there is an ECG machine ready to hand, do an ECG trace. Unless the patient has COPD, unrestricted oxygen should be given; if the patient has COPD, give 24% oxygen. If heart failure seems likely, give 40 mg furosemide iv: it will do little or no harm in the other conditions listed above. If there is wheezing, give 2.5 mg salbutamol by nebuliser. If you think the patient has a tension pneumothorax, inserting a large-bore needle or cannula through the chest wall can be life-saving. The next step is to transfer the patient urgently to medical care or to the A&E department. If you think the patient has stridor, they need to see an ear, nose and throat (ENT) surgeon very urgently. If this is impossible, send the patient to the A&E department.

Stridor

Stridor is a harsh type of noisy breathing caused by obstruction of a large airway (bronchus, trachea, larynx). Patients can deteriorate very rapidly and die. Although it may be confused with wheezing, the noise is generated at the site of the obstruction. Careful examination will usually resolve the issue. The emergency treatment is to give heliox and to transfer to an ENT surgeon, as an emergency tracheostomy may be needed. Give heliox by facemask during transfer of the patient. If the situation is very severe, and especially if heliox does not help, placing a wide-bore cannula through the cricothyroid membrane can be life-saving. You will probably not feel confident to attempt a tracheotomy, and in any case, a tracheotomy kit will probably not be available.

Tension pneumothorax

A one-way valve mechanism results in a progressive rise in pleural pressure. The mediastinum will move to the opposite side (trachea deviates, apex beat moves). This impairs venous return to the heart and the potential for cardiopulmonary collapse. Delayed treatment is associated with a high mortality, so, if you encounter a tension pneumothorax, you must treat it immediately by pushing a large-bore needle or cannula through the chest wall, which will decompress the hemithorax. Having done this, the patient should receive oxygen and be transferred quickly to the acute medical service for insertion of a chest drain.

Oxygen therapy

Oxygen is essential for life. Oxygen therapy is given to acutely ill patients who have hypoxaemia from pneumonia, acute severe asthma, left ventricular failure and exacerbations of chronic obstructive airways disease. These patients will be dealt with by the emergency medical services in hospital, and such patients should not be staying under the care of old age psychiatrists.

Oxygen is also given in two other settings: first, for symptomatic treatment of patients with chronic lung disease, and second, as life-prolonging treatment for patients with persistent hypoxaemia from chronic lung disease.

Patients with chronic lung disease such as chronic obstructive airways disease get symptomatic relief from oxygen, which they may use as and when required, to relieve breathlessness. Patients may be provided with a cylinder of oxygen at home which they may take usually via a face-mask. This type of oxygen therapy does not improve survival.

For patients with chronic severe hypoxaemia, prolonged oxygen therapy for over 15 hours per day improves survival. These patients should have been assessed by a chest physician for their suitability for long-term oxygen therapy (LTOT). Blood gases estimations confirming persistent hypoxaemia, taken when the patient is clinically stable, are used to determine the appropriateness for long-term oxygen therapy. Oxygen is usually provided from oxygen concentrators which are installed in patients' homes. Oxygen is usually delivered via nasal specula to improve comfort and compliance.

Some patients with cognitive impairment may be poorly compliant with oxygen therapy. For those who are acutely ill, good-nursing care is needed to enhance compliance. For those patients using oxygen symptomatically there is no imperative to enforce treatment. Patients considered for long-term oxygen therapy will have been assessed to determine whether they are likely to be compliant with treatment. As benefit is seen only for those patients using oxygen for over 15 hours per day, if they are not compliant then therapy is ineffective and should be discontinued.

Nebuliser therapy

Nebulisers are widely used in emergency and acute treatment of asthma and chronic obstructive airways disease. Large doses of drugs can be delivered as an aerosol in a short period of time. Nebulisers are also used as domiciliary therapy for patients with severe symptoms from chronic lung disease. Chest physicians usually assess this group of patients for their suitability for long-term nebuliser treatment. Most patients with chronic lung disease are managed with standard metered-dose inhalers with or without spacer devices. Breath-activated and dry-powder devices are also available, which are easier to use. Nebulisers have the advantage that they are not operator-dependent, but would seldom be used because of poor inhaler technique. If patients with cognitive impairment cannot take inhaled therapy, they can be assisted by nursing staff. Oral preparations of beta-sympathomimetics are also available for those unable to use inhalers.

Inhaled steroids are used to control asthma and prevent symptoms. They are also used in some patients with severe COPD. If patients are unable to manage inhalers, low-dose oral prednisolone can be considered as an alternative. A chest physician or geriatrician can advise on alternative treatments.

COMA/SLEEP/ALTERED MENTAL STATE

What we refer to by this section heading is 'a disturbance in either the level or the content of consciousness'. Thus, there is considerable overlap in the differential diagnoses for mild confusional states, delirium, dementia and coma. As this book is targeted at old age psychiatrists, we make only passing reference here (and elsewhere in the book) to the first three of these.

Consciousness

It is easy to get into difficulties when discussing consciousness, and to stray from neuroscience into the philosophy of the mind. Even its definition is difficult, although, like a bespoke suit, you can recognise it without seeing the label. Despite the difficulties in definition, there is relatively good agreement about at least some of the components of consciousness:

(1) Awareness;

(2) Self-awareness;

(3) Temporality (sense of now and sense of time);

(4) Memory;

(5) Feelings (emotions, desires);

(6) Intentions;

(7) Expectations;

(8) Thoughts (beliefs, ideas, reason, inner imagery).

Being alert (level of arousal) is necessary for the proper expression of these factors: consciousness does not just happen – it takes work. Recently, orexin-producing neurons have been implicated in the maintenance of wakefulness, and they are inhibited only by neurons active during sleep (a genetically determined orexin deficiency is associated with narcolepsy).

Neuroanatomy of arousal

The critical regulator of arousal and alertness is the reticular formation, two sausage-shaped, tangled collections of neurons running through the core of the brainstem, from the thalamus to the medulla. These neurons are ideally located to integrate all sensory information passing from the body to the brain. Neurons here do not seem to have precise specificity for components of sensory information, but rather to the degree of such sensory input. A key component of the reticular formation is the reticular activating system (RAS), which lies mainly in the pons. Acetylcholine is the main neurotrammsmitter of the RAS. Axons of the RAS project to other brainstem areas, the thalamus and many cortical areas, especially the basal forebrain. Activity of the RAS is necessary to maintain wakefulness (dopaminergic pathways from the ventral tegmentum play a role in its regulation). As sleep is entered and progresses, RAS activity declines, only to become hyperactive during rapid eye movement (REM) sleep. This latter state activates the neuronal firing associated with dreaming by internal activation of the visual system and other cortical sensory and emotional areas.

During REM sleep, other neurons are activated which suppress motor output, resulting in near-paralysis. The serotonin and noradrenaline projection systems of the reticular formation are also relatively inactive during sleep. These neurons project widely to the cortex, normally focusing attention and allowing memory formation. Thus, the cognitive activities of REM sleep lack internal coordination, which contributes to the often fantastic and bizarre nature of dreams.

Sleep

Sleep is a very primitive biological drive of, as yet, unknown function. It appears that even insects sleep in a way similar to humans and display similar types of changes during aging. They require 10–11 hours per day and show similar consequences of sleep deprivation to humans. Interestingly, there is a mutation of the potassium channel in fruit-flies that allows them to require only 2–3 hours of sleep per 24 hours, and they are resistant to the effects of sleep deprivation. Marine mammals seem to be able to sleep one hemisphere at a time. The precise control of sleep is not yet understood, and no single neuroanatomical area is responsible for sleep. There seems to be a balance between sleep-promoting (γ-aminobutyric acid (GABA)-ergic and galaninergic) neurons in the ventral preoptic hypothalamus and wake-promoting (hypocretin) neurons in the lateral hypothalamus. Fine adjustment of the sleep–wake cycle seems to be a function of the suprachiasmatic nucleus (serotonergic). Adenosine seems important in reducing arousal and alertness (caffeine and theophylline interfere with this). It seems that sleep patterns established in infancy are strongly related to those experienced in later life.

Sleep usually progresses through stages, with characteristic changes in the EEG. During stage 1 (light sleep), we drift in and out of sleep and can be woken easily. Our eyes move very slowly and muscle activity slows. People woken from stage 1 sleep often remember fragmented visual images. Many also experience sudden muscle contractions called hypnic myoclonia, often preceded by a sensation of starting to fall. When stage 2 sleep is entered, eye movements stop and electrical activity slows, with occasional bursts of rapid waves called sleep spindles. In stage 3, extremely slow brain waves (delta waves) begin to appear, interspersed with smaller, faster waves. By stage 4, the brain produces delta waves almost exclusively. It is very difficult to wake someone during stages 3 and 4, which together are called deep sleep. There is no eye movement or muscle activity. People woken during deep sleep do not adjust immediately, and often feel groggy and disoriented for several minutes after they wake up.

When we move into REM sleep, the respiratory rate increases and becomes irregular and shallow; the eyes jerk rapidly in various directions, and limb muscles become temporarily paralysed. The heart rate increases and blood pressure rises, and men develop penile erections. When people awaken during REM sleep, they often describe bizarre and illogical stories (dreams). The first REM sleep period usually occurs about 70–90 min after falling asleep. A complete sleep cycle takes 90–110 min on average. The first sleep cycles each night contain relatively short REM periods and long periods of deep sleep. As the night progresses, REM sleep periods increase in length while deep sleep decreases. By morning, people spend nearly all their sleep time in stages 1, 2 and REM.

People woken after sleeping for more than a few minutes are usually unable to recall the last few minutes before they fell asleep. This sleep-related form of amnesia is the reason that people often forget telephone calls or conversations they have had in the middle of the night. It also explains why people often do not remember alarm-clocks ringing in the morning if they do not get up immediately after turning them off.

People who are under general anaesthesia or in a coma do not produce the complex, active brain-wave patterns seen in normal sleep. Instead, the brain electrical activity is very slow and weak, sometimes barely detectable.

How much sleep is necessary?

The amount of sleep needed depends on many factors, including age. Infants generally require about 16 hours a day. Most adults find that 7–8 hours each night is sufficient, although some people may need as few as 5 hours or as many as 10 hours. The amount of sleep a person needs increases if he/she has been deprived of sleep in previous days. Getting too little sleep creates a 'sleep debt', which must be repaid. We know that sleep deprivation is dangerous. Sleep-deprived people perform badly on tasks of hand–eye coordination (as badly as, or worse than, those who are intoxicated with alcohol). Further, sleep deprivation magnifies the effects of alcohol. Sleep deprivation impairs the ability to drive safely.

People tend to sleep more lightly and for shorter time spans as they get older, although they generally need about the same amount of sleep in total as they needed in early adulthood. About half of all people over the age of

65 years complain of sleeping problems, such as insomnia: deep sleep stages in many elderly people often become very short or may cease entirely. This may be a normal part of aging, or it may result from medical problems, medications and other treatments for those problems.

Feeling drowsy during the daytime, even during boring activities, implies lack of sleep. Falling asleep within 5 minutes of lying down indicates a more marked lack of sleep, or even a sleep disorder. Microsleeps are another mark of sleep deprivation, and often, people are not aware that they are experiencing them.

Microsleeps

Microsleeps are brief, unintended episodes of loss of attention associated with events such as blank stare, head snapping and prolonged eye closure, which may occur when a person is fatigued but trying to stay awake to perform a monotonous task such as driving a car, reading a book, listening to a lecture or watching a computer screen.

Episodes last from a few seconds to several minutes, and often, the person is not aware that a microsleep has occurred. Microsleeps may take place with the eyes open. During a microsleep, a person does not respond to external information: a person will not see a red traffic light or notice a bend in the road. Microsleeps are commonest in the early hours of the morning and in the mid-afternoon hour. As the sleep debt increases, microsleep frequency also increases.

Sleep disorders

Complaints regarding aspects of sleeping are extremely common, especially among older people (30–50%). Sleep disorders can be classified into three broad groups:

(1)   Insomnias;

(2)   Parasomnias;

(3)   Hypersomnias.

Insomnias

Complaints include changes in the pattern of falling asleep, frequent waking, early waking and unrefreshing sleep. Insomnia may be primary (not explained by some other condition or treatment) or secondary to some other disorder (medications, pain, depression, restless legs, etc.). In addition, some people feel that they do not get enough sleep, when investigation for a sleep disorder suggests that they do have sufficient sleep (pseudo-insomnia). Usually, the history and examination is sufficient to identify the likely underlying cause. Hypnic headache (page 119) causes abrupt waking with a severe pulsating headache: it is a condition seen almost only in older people, usually women. Drugs commonly associated with insomnia include:

(1)   Alcohol;

(2)   Anticholinergics;

(3)   β-Adrenorceptor antagonists;

(4)   Caffeine (in coffee);

(5)   Theophylline (in tea);

(6)   Methyl-dihydroxyphenylalanine (DOPA);

(7)   Serotonin-selective reuptake inhibitors (SSRIs);

(8)   Monoamine oxidase inhibitors (MAOIs);

(9)   Sympathomimetics;

(10) Cimetidine.

Approaching a patient with difficulties initiating and maintaining sleep

The first thing to realise is that patients often overestimate sleep complaints. The history is aimed at elucidating the precise nature and extent of the problem. What is the person's 'usual' sleep pattern? Do people nap in the daytime? Is the total sleep over 24 hours adequate? Are there problems of sleep onset and/or awakenings? How often do they awaken and why (e.g. pain, dreams, anxiety)? What medications are being taken and could any of these affect sleep? Are there any features of depression? Is there evidence from a witness (spouse, carer, nurse)?

Many somatic disorders interfere with sleep, so you need information about the past medical and surgical history. Similarly, a complete physical examination is required unless the cause is obvious. The screening investigations we list earlier (page 5) should suffice at this stage.

Many complaints of insomnia are transient and often related to a significant life-event, including being in hospital. Usually, patients can be reassured without needing to prescribe hypnotics. You may also need to consider moving a noisy patient to a side-room: hypnotics are not the treatment for another person shouting all night. Chronicity may develop if the sleeping problem is allowed to persist for more than 3–4 weeks, so temporary use of hypnotics may be needed.

Conventionally, insomnia lasting more than 3 weeks is referred to as chronic insomnia. It is necessary to exclude somatic causes (especially pain, breathlessness, need to pass urine, etc.) and medications, as for acute insomnia, before attributing it to a psychological or psychiatric disorder. If there is a psychiatric cause, the intervention should be directed towards that. Continued use of hypnotics should be avoided, as they rapidly cease to be effective and induce dependence, making their withdrawal difficult: the BNF gives instructions on how to withdraw benzodiazepines safely. With recurrent sleepless nights, short courses of treatment may be warranted. Short-acting agents (e.g. zopliclone) may be most useful for sleep-onset problems, although they may be associated with early-morning insomnia and anterograde amnesia in higher doses. Slow-onset and sustained-action agents (e.g. temazepam) help little with sleep onset but reduce awakenings. If longer-term use is unavoidable, we have found it helpful to give a benzodiazepine for 1–2 weeks, alternating with another agent (e.g. clomethiazole). Hypnic headache is responsive to treatment with lithium.

Parasomnias

These are non-epileptic phenomena associated with sleep. Generally, they are benign. Such phenomena include:

(1)   Myoclonic jerks;

(2)   Nightmares;

(3)   Night terrors;

(4)   Talking in sleep (somniloquy);

(5)   Teeth grinding (bruxism);

(6)   Sleep paralysis;

(7)   Sleep walking (somnambulism);

(8)   REM sleep behaviour disorder (RBD).

The onset of sleepwalking (which occurs during deep sleep) in older people suggests a psychiatric disorder (e.g. dementia) or an effect of medication. Benzodiazepines suppress deep sleep and may ameliorate sleepwalking.

Hypersomnias

Hypersomnia may be secondary to some other disorder (medications, Parkinson's disease, dystrophia myotonica, brain tumour, stroke, head injury, thyroid disease) or it may present as a primary disorder. These primary disorders comprise a number of conditions, which usually require specialist investigation for correct diagnosis. They include:

(1)   Obstructive sleep apnoeas (OSAs);

(2)   Central sleep apnoeas (CSAs).

OSA is usually associated with profound snoring with increasing ventilatory effort, or even cessation of breathing, with brief arousals from sleep. Such patients may complain of early-morning headache. These patients are usually best referred to someone with an interest in sleep disorders (often a neurologist or respiratory physician) for diagnosis.

CSA is associated with disorders affecting the lower brainstem, with loss of automatic breathing, particularly during sleep (Ondine's curse). Many CSAs are usually seen only in young people, and are not discussed here. Generally, if you suspect one of these, refer to a clinician with an interest in sleep disorders. Other conditions you may encounter include:

(1)   Narcolepsy (Gélineau's syndrome);

(2)   Nocturnal hypoventilation (usually with some neuromuscular disorder);

(3)   Idiopathic hypersomnolence.

Although rare, narcolepsy does present in old age. Symptoms include daytime sleepiness, irresistible desires for sleep and brief naps (which refresh the person). Cataplexy (transient episodic weakness or paralysis) is common and may cause (injurious) falls, often precipitated by strong emotion (laughter, anger). Sleep paralysis occurs in the transition between sleep and waking, often with an inability even to speak. Hypnagogic and hypnapompic hallucinations may be regarded as dreaming whilst awake.

Disorders of diminished consciousness (stupor and coma)

Full consciousness requires the pontomesencephalic tegmentum of at least one-half of the brainstem and the ipsilateral diencephalon and some of the ipsilateral cerebral hemisphere. Consciousness is preserved (provided that breathing and blood pressure can be supported) without the spinal cord, medulla, caudal part of the pons, cerebellum, tectum, lemnisci and cranial nerve nuclei. It is also preserved with any two of the four cerebral lobes or with one hemisphere (with a small part of the other). Consciousness lies on a continuum which can be stratified into ten levels:

(1) Convulsions;

(2) Mania;

(3) Euphoria;

(4) Insomnia;

(5) Hyperalertness;

(6) Alertness;

(7) Somnolence;

(8) Sopor (obtundation);

(9) Stupor;

(10) Coma.

In this subsection, we are concerned only with the final three levels. Patients who present in this state will have a medical explanation, rather than a neurological one, in 70–80% of cases. Such patients represent a medical emergency. In the very late stages of many dementias, patients predictably lapse into unconsciousness, and such patients should be managed with palliative measures only. It is common to assign a Glasgow Coma Scale score (GCS; Table 4.1), which has prognostic significance, particularly after head injury or cardiorespiratory arrest. The scoring is usually repeated at intervals to monitor the course.

Immediate measures in an unconscious patient

(1) Clear and maintain the airway;

(2) Check pulse, blood pressure, temperature (treat profound hypotension or dysrhythmia) and pupils (size, symmetry);

(3) Insert an intravenous line and stick test blood for glucose (send blood for FBC, glucose and electrolytes; blood is usually also sent for liver and thyroid function);

(4) Give thiamine, 100 mg iv, followed by 50 ml of 50% glucose (if not hyperglycaemic on stick testing);

Table 4.1 The Glasgow Coma Scale

Eyes open	
Never	1
To pain	2
To verbal stimuli	3
Spontaneously	4
Best verbal response	
No response	1
Incomprehensible sounds	2
Inappropriate words	3
Disoriented and converses	4
Oriented and converses	5
Best motor response	
No response	1
Extension (decerebrate rigidity)	2
Flexion abnormal (decorticate rigidity)	3
Localises pain	4
Obeys	5
Total	__ (range 3–14)

(5)   If the patient has received opioids, give 2 mg of naloxone iv (up to a maximum of 10 mg);

(6)   Catheterise to measure urine output;

(7)   Assess the GCS;

(8)   Assess responsiveness to pain (press styloid processes, supraorbital foramina, sternum or between the eyes and note the response (arousal, decerebrate posturing, decorticate posturing, asymmetrical movements, no response)).

Soporose patients respond to verbal stimuli but are drowsy, slow and disoriented. Stuporose patients respond transiently to vigorous stimuli only. The comatose are unarousable but may exhibit abnormal postures.

Examining the unconscious patient

In essence, the objective is to differentiate CNS causes of unconsciousness from other (usually metabolic) causes. If trauma is suspected, immobilise the neck. The essential information, some of which will already be available, includes:

(1) Vital signs (pulse, blood pressure, temperature);

(2) Breathing pattern;

(3) Pupils (size, symmetry);

(4) Neck stiffness;

(5) Oculocephalic response;

(6) Posture;

(7) Deep tendon reflexes;

(8) Myoclonus;

(9) Evidence of head injury (bruising, boggy swelling).

Normal breathing, coughing, swallowing, yawning and hiccups all suggest that the cranial nerves IX, X and XII are functioning and that the pontomedullary reticular formation and cervical and upper thoracic spinal cord are intact. Blinking or tonic eyelid closure shows the cranial nerves V and VII to be intact. Random, slow deviations of the eyes to the sides (lost before the oculocephalic responses are lost) show intact cranial nerves III, IV and VI and also the frontopontine pathway that drives them. Because of the positions of the relevant nuclei, these features show the entire pons and medulla to be intact. If random, spontaneous movements of all four limbs are seen, this implies unimpaired pyramidal tracts all the way to the sacral segments of the spinal cord. If all these signs are present, a large structural lesion is eliminated as a cause for the coma.

Other features suggesting a CNS cause are increased blood pressure, irregular breathing, asymmetrical pupils, neck stiffness, asymmetrical (or absent) oculocephalic response, abnormal posture and asymmetrical deep tendon reflexes. Bruising in a 'panda distribution' may indicate a frontal bone fracture: bruising behind the mastoid (Battle's sign) suggests fracture of the base of the skull.

A non-CNS cause is suggested by decreased blood pressure, regular breathing, normally reactive pupils, intact oculocephalic response, symmetrical posture, absence of neck stiffness, symmetrical deep tendon reflexes and myoclonic jerks.

If the blood pressure is high and the pulse is slow, think of raised intracranial pressure: this may be associated with asymmetrically dilated pupils, and the ocular fundus may show loss of venous pulsation and/or signs of papilloedema. Regular, rapid, deep breathing suggests metabolic acidosis (uraemia, diabetes, ethylene glycol), although it may also be seen with mid-brain lesions (central neurogenic hyperpnoea). Reduced rate and depth of ventilation suggest drug overdose or a medullary lesion. Cheyne–Stokes breathing (cyclically increased and decreased rate and depth of breathing) occurs in both metabolic and CNS causes of coma. Irregular (ataxic) breathing signifies cerebellar or pontine haemorrhage, medullary infarction or severe meningitis.

Mild asymmetry of the pupils (1 mm) is normal. Greater asymmetry suggests a CNS cause or previous eye surgery. Small, pinpoint pupils suggest narcotic overdose or pontine haemorrhage: note that small pupils are common in normal older people and in those on treatment for glaucoma. Bilaterally fixed, dilated pupils suggest cholinergic poisoning (atropine, scopolamine), bilateral tentorial herniation or cerebral anoxia.

Neck stiffness is a feature of meningitis or subarachnoid haemorrhage; note that in older people, neck stiffness may reflect degenerative disease of the cervical spine. Do not assess for neck stiffness or test the oculocephalic responses if you suspect head and neck trauma.

Oculocephalic responses

The oculocephalic response is tested by holding the eyelids open and rapidly rotating the head to each side in turn. If the brainstem reflexes are intact, the eyes will move in the direction opposite to that of the rotation. Thus, a normal response indicates that the brainstem is normal between cranial nerve III (oculomotor) and cranial nerve VIII (vestibuloauditory), suggesting that the cause of coma does not lie in the brainstem, at least between these levels. An abnormal response implies a severe brainstem disorder or a 'metabolic cause'. If the result of this test is equivocal, or the test cannot be done owing to suspected neck trauma, try caloric testing. Before doing the test, inspect the external auditory meatus and remove any wax, look for otitis and a perforated drum (coma can arise from extension of middle-ear infection into the brain). The test is done by irrigating the ear canal with 5–20 ml of iced water. This suppresses the ipsilateral vestibular labyrinth, and the normal response is for the eyes to deviate towards the side of irrigation. An abnormal response is for no movement to take place. Only two disorders make interpretation difficult: sedative drug overdose and hypothermia. In these two settings, the patient needs to be tested repeatedly over several days.

Posture

The decerebrate posture is characterised by extended and internally rotated arms and legs extended in plantar flexion. Symmetrical decerebrate posturing indicates severe brainstem damage or a 'metabolic' coma. The decorticate posture is characterised by arm flexion and leg extension in plantar flexion. Symmetrical decorticoid posturing is seen with bilateral hemisphere lesions. Asymmetrical posturing with movement on the other side suggests a CNS cause for the coma. Decorticate posturing on one side and decerebrate posturing on the other also points to a CNS cause.

Opisthotonos

This means 'bowed-backwards', and arises from contraction of the powerful spinal extensor muscles. It occurs with meningeal irritation (blood, inflammation), bilateral decerebrate rigidity, rabies, tetanus, strychnine poisoning, hysteria and catatonic schizophrenia.

Internal herniations of the brain

The most common causes of these are cerebral contusions, haematomas, abscesses, neoplasms and cerebral oedema. These all cause raised intracranial pressure and internal shifts or herniations of the brain to compress tissue elsewhere, usually the diencephalon and brainstem. The herniation occurs under the fixed structures of the falx cerebri and the tentorium cerebelli. Sometimes, herniation of the cerebellum and medulla can take place into the foramen magnum: this causes quadriplegia and apnoea. Most often, it is the cingulate gyrus that herniates under the falx, compressing the ipsilateral anterior cerebral artery, which may cause impaired consciousness and also infarction of the medial hemispheric wall dorsal to the corpus callosum. The posterior cerebral artery may also be compressed as it crosses the free edge of the falx, resulting in infarction of the medial temporo-occipital region, commonly causing contralateral homonymous hemianopia and/or prosopagnosia. Transtentorial herniation is of the uncus and/or the parahippocampal gyrus. This compresses the third cranial nerve and the mid-brain, thereby causing ipsilateral pupillary dilatation and suppressed consciousness. As the herniation progresses, both oculomotor nerves become compressed and the pupils are dilated and fixed. Death follows without immediate neurosurgical intervention.

Disorders such as cerebral oedema, encephalitis, metabolic conditions (uraemia, hepatic coma), subdural haematomas, hydrocephalus, multiple metastases or abscesses and brain haemorrhage may result in bilateral transtentorial herniation. The resulting ring of swollen tissue forms a ligature around the mid-brain. This is commonly followed by pontine haemorrhage and death.

Information from the history

When available, the history often points to the likely cause of coma. Important points are:

(1) Onset (sudden = haemorrhage or infarct, gradual = toxic and metabolic);

(2) Neurological disease (epilepsy, headache, diplopia, vertigo, numbness, weakness, ataxia);

(3) Recent trauma;

(4) Medications;

(5) Psychiatric history (depression, suicide attempts).

Diagnosis and management

The diagnosis of coma will usually be clear, but you should also consider akinetic mutism, catatonia and the locked-in syndrome. After the above assessment, which can be done very quickly, the likelihood of a CNS or non-CNS cause should be apparent. Do not forget that a non-CNS diagnosis will always be more likely in the absence of head trauma.

Common medical causes

(1) Hypoxia (cardiac arrest, respiratory failure, sedative drug or opioid overdose);

(2) Drug overdose (sedative drugs, insulin, opioids – reversible with naloxone, benzodiazepines – reversible with flumazenil, barbiturates, alcohol);

(3) Diabetes (hypoglycaemia, HONK, ketoacidosis);

(4) Severe electrolyte abnormalities;

(5) Uraemia;

(6) Liver failure;

(7) Heat stroke.

If you suspect opioid overdose, give naloxone and note the response. If you suspect benzodiazepine overdose, try flumazenil, but be aware that it can induce withdrawal symptoms in those dependent on benzodiazepines: read about this drug in the BNF before using it. Except in patients in the advanced stages of neurodegenerative disorders, in whom the lapse into coma should be predictable and be predicted, all these patients need urgent referral to the acute medical service for further management.

CNS causes

(1)   Head injury;

(2)   Subdural haematoma;

(3)   Intracerebral bleed/subarachnoid haemorrhage;

(4)   Cerebral herniation;

(5)   Posterior fossa mass;

(6)   Brainstem infarction/haemorrhage;

(7)   Cerebral metastases/abscesses;

(8)   Meningitis/encephalitis;

(9)   Non-convulsive status epilepticus.

All of these require urgent transfer to the acute medical service for further assessment and management. If cerebral herniation is a serious possibility, give mannitol (0.5–1 g/kg body weight over 20–30 min) before transferring for further assessment and management, ideally by neurosurgeons. An emergency CT scan will be required. The further management will ideally be in the intensive-care unit.

Akinetic mutism

The patient appears alert and can follow the examiner with their eyes. The sleep–wake cycle persists but there is no voluntary spontaneous motor activity or vocalisations. It is associated with bilateral lesions in the frontal lobes, thalamus and the mid-brain reticular formation (which may impair consciousness). This is generally considered as part of the persistent vegetative state.

Locked-in syndrome

Lesions of the upper tegmentum of the ventral pons or mid-brain cause deafferentation of the lower cranial nerves and the peripheral motor system, usually at the level of the facial nuclei. Lateral gaze is sometimes also lost. The patients are self-aware but can communicate only through eye movements ('a corpse with living eyes').

CONSTIPATION

Normal bowel movements occur between three times daily and three times weekly. The Latin origin of the word constipation relates to the consistency of the stool: it is hard. However, the term is now used also to refer to infrequent bowel movements regardless of consistency, arbitrarily fewer than three times per week. Constipation, in most cases, has one of four mechanisms:

(1)   Delayed transit;

(2)   Outlet obstruction (mechanical, pelvic floor dysfunction);

(3)   Decreased awareness of 'the call to stool';

(4)   Unfulfilled expectations (cultural).

Everybody experiences constipation from time to time, but constipation is a particularly common complaint among older people. Almost half of the older population in the UK take laxatives on a regular basis, although not all necessarily need them. Treatment is usually needed only if the problem is persistent. Associated symptoms can include:

(1)   Need to strain at stool;

(2)   Need to assist evacuation digitally;

(3)   Abdominal bloating and distension;

(4)   Rectal fullness;

(5)   Left lower quadrant pain;

(6)   Generalised discomfort.

If these symptoms arise in the setting of weight loss, anaemia or other evidence of bleeding in the bowel, there is a high likelihood of colonic cancer.

Abdominal distension should raise concerns about mechanical obstruction, which may be caused by neoplasm but also by other local pathology, such as rectal prolapse, rectal intussusception, sigmoid volvulus, strictures and external compression by a pelvic mass.

Colonic motility can decline, and the colon can distend after surgery and also with other severe systemic illnesses, with electrolyte disturbances and after the administration of a number of medications (especially opiates, calcium channel blockers and anticholinergics). In the absence of other pointers in the history, in an old age psychiatry setting, drugs should be reviewed as possible underlying causes, particularly:

(1) Anticholinergics (antidepressants, antipsychotics, anti-Parkinson's disease, antihistamines);

(2) Diuretics;

(3) Iron preparations;

(4) Sympathomimetics (ephedrine, salbutamol, terbutaline);

(5) Antacids (especially those containing aluminium);

(6) Antihypertensives (ACEIs, calcium channel blockers);

(7) NSAIDs.

Sometimes, constipation can be severe and faecal loading can follow, with bypass and leakage of liquid stool around the solid faecal masses: incontinence of this liquid stool may occur and may easily be misdiagnosed and mistreated as diarrhoea.

Treatment

If medication is thought to be the major aetiological factor, you need to review whether the drug(s) in question are required or not. Regardless, all patients need an examination of the abdomen including a rectal examination (see page 56). You should also check blood electrolytes and calcium.

Patients thought to have some form of lower bowel obstruction require further investigation, and such patients should be referred elsewhere for this. If an obstructive lesion is unlikely, then the treatment should be focused on the problem, namely constipation. General advice should include ensuring adequate hydration and physical activity. This alone will usually be inadequate, in which case bulking agents including bran should be considered. An inadequate response might prompt the associated use of either a stool softener or glycerine suppository. If the stool is not especially hard and the complaint of constipation continues, a stimulant laxative such as senna or bisacodyl is appropriate. Lactulose should not be given as it is relatively ineffective, relatively unpleasant to take, messy to administer and expensive.

If an adequate response has not been achieved using the above measures, an osmotic laxative (we suggest Movicol®) is usually effective. If the response is poor, micro-enemas or phosphate enemas can be considered. Occasional patients resist all the above measures to induce defaecation and become faecally loaded. In this case, the patient needs to be re-evaluated for the possibility of an obstructive lesion. People unable to expel hard stool may well be able to expel soft stool, so stool softening is important in these patients. You should also consider requesting further advice (geriatrician, gastroenterologist or colorectal surgeon) at this stage. Large volumes of polyethylene glycol-containing laxatives (e.g. Klean-Prep®) will almost always be effective (eventually!) as solid stool also dissolves, although this approach can precipitate incontinence (sometimes massive) of large volumes of liquid stool. Rarely, surgery may ultimately be needed, and a variety of approaches are taken (e.g. posterior anal myotomy, resection) depending on the underlying disorder.

COUGH

Cough is a beneficial reflex designed to protect the respiratory tract. It is induced by afferent mechanical, thermal and chemical stimuli triggering receptors in the larynx, tracheobronchial tree, pleura and diaphragm. Causes of cough include:

(1)   Upper respiratory infection (often viral);

(2)   Lower respiratory infection;

(3)   Smoking;

(4)   Asthma;

(5)   COPD;

(6)   Sinusitis;

(7)   Gastro-oesophageal reflux disease (GORD);

(8)   Swallowing disorders (aspiration);

(9)   Bronchiectasis;

(10) ACEI treatment;

(11) Heart failure;

(12) Lung cancer.

History

The history should determine whether the cough is acute, recurrent or chronic. Is there sneezing, earache, runny eyes and nose or sore throat? You should also determine whether or not the cough is productive of sputum or blood. Is the cough worse at night than in the daytime? Is coughing induced by changing position? Is coughing occurring in association with swallowing problems? Are there constitutional features to suggest infection such as feeling inappropriately cold or shivering? Does the patient feel hot? Weakness, malaise and muscle aching suggest a systemic inflammatory response associated with significant infection.

Acute cough is usually infective in origin, most often viral: has there been an outbreak of coughing on the ward? If the sputum is thick and purulent, the cause is usually acute bronchitis, pneumonia, bronchiectasis, lung abscess and (occasionally) chronic bronchitis. Cough induced by position change is often caused by chronic bronchitis, lung abscess, bronchiectasis, GORD and endobronchial tumour. If the cough is worse at night, think of GORD and asthma.

Examination

Check pulse, blood pressure and temperature. Examine the respiratory and cardiovascular systems. Assess swallowing (page 193) if aspiration is a possibility.

Investigations

Most mild upper-respiratory infections require no investigations. Blood should be sent for urea and electrolytes and white cell count. Send sputum for culture. Sputum can also be sent for cytology if the cough is chronic or if there are features suggesting lung cancer: do not send it for cytology if the sputum is purulent. Check peak expiratory flow rate and spirometry if there is any suggestion of asthma or chronic airflow limitation (asthma, COPD). A chest radiograph is indicated if:

(1)   A lower respiratory infection is suspected;

(2)   There is haemoptysis;

(3)   There is new cough not explained by infection.

A chronic cough with a normal chest radiograph suggests asthma. If the diagnosis remains unclear, refer for help: a bronchoscopy is likely to be needed.

Management

Coughs associated with swallowing problems require a detailed swallowing assessment (page 193). An acute cough with sneezing, sore throat, runny eyes and runny nose strongly suggests a viral upper respiratory infection. This is generally self-limiting, and antibiotics are not indicated. Occasionally, mycoplasma infections can present like this, although there will usually also be physical signs of lower respiratory infection on examination or chest radiograph. These infections should be treated with erythromycin or a tetracycline. Some viral infections cause severe systemic symptoms (e.g. influenza), and older people may become severely ill and may develop secondary bacterial pneumonia. It is recommended that all people of the age of 65 years or over should receive annual immunisation against influenza. Further, antiviral drugs (e.g. zanamivir) may be given to patients within 48 hours of the onset of symptoms of influenza during an influenza outbreak.

A lower respiratory infection will be indicated by a more severe illness, fever and purulent sputum. Patients will usually need parenteral fluids if the illness is severe. Treatment should be indicated by the results of sputum culture. 'Blind' treatment before the results of culture are available will usually be on the basis of local hospital guidelines. The antibiotic should be changed to as narrow-spectrum an agent as possible when culture results are available. A prompt response to the appropriate antibiotic is expected: if this does not happen, refer the patient to the geriatrics service. For most of the other causes of cough listed (and many others that we have not listed), the help of the geriatrics service will be required.

Dehydration

The usual clinical signs of dehydration such as loss of skin turgor, sunken eyes and dry mouth may be present in normal elderly subjects, and are thus unreliable. Symptoms of postural hypotension may be present. Supine hypotension and tachycardia may be present in severe cases. Acute weight loss can be measured, and weight loss in kilograms is equivalent to litres of fluid lost. In hospitalised elderly subjects, fluid balance charts are important in at-risk patients to avoid dehydration.

Venesection for plasma urea, creatinine and electrolytes is necessary. Urine output monitoring is required to avoid pre-renal kidney failure.

Replacement fluid depends on the type of fluid loss. With predominant water loss, dehydration is accompanied by hypernatraemia. With isotonic fluid loss, sodium levels are normal. Management depends on the severity of fluid loss. Drugs aggravating dehydration, such as diuretics, should be stopped. If mild dehydration is present, oral rehydration can be done using water with or without salt supplementation. Intravenous fluids are required for more severe dehydration, and transfer to a medical ward may be necessary. Subcutaneous fluid replacement can be used in long-term care settings to maintain fluid intake.

Terminal dehydration is seen at the end of many illnesses. Food and fluid intake generally diminish in the terminal stage of illness. The traditional hospice view is that once a patient loses interest in food and fluid it need not be given. It is also argued that fluids increase secretions and excretion, which can be more inconvenient for the patient. There is no evidence that rehydration makes the patient more comfortable. Indications for hydration would be to relieve symptoms, for example if a patient feels dry despite good mouth care.

DIABETES MELLITUS

Diabetes mellitus is a metabolic disorder producing chronic hyperglycaemia and associated with disturbances of carbohydrate, fat and protein metabolism. It arises either through an absolute deficiency of insulin – type 1 or insulin-dependent diabetes mellitus (IDDM) – or through a combination of resistance to insulin action coupled with an inadequate compensatory insulin secretory response – type 2, maturity-onset diabetes or non-insulin-dependent diabetes mellitus (NIDDM). Diabetes mellitus is common in old age (10% prevalence) and is usually non-insulin-dependent, although many patients will have their diabetes controlled with insulin therapy. Most cases of diabetes mellitus are primary, i.e. not associated with other diseases, but diabetes may also occur secondary to other conditions, e.g. chronic pancreatitis, or conditions associated with the secretion of hormones antagonistic to insulin, e.g. Cushing's disease, or be associated with acromegaly or drugs such as glucocorticoids.

Diabetes is associated with both immediate metabolic disturbances and the development of long-term complications. The metabolic disturbances, which can be life-threatening if untreated, include ketoacidosis, which develops in insulin-dependent diabetic patients, non-ketotic hyperglycaemia and lactic acidosis.

The long-term complications are related to microvascular disease, namely retinopathy, neuropathy and nephropathy, and to macrovascular disease (i.e. atherosclerosis), causing ischaemic heart disease, peripheral vascular disease and stroke.

The diagnosis of diabetes is made by demonstrating the presence of hyperglycaemia. In the presence of symptoms, a random venous plasma or capillary blood glucose greater than 11.1 mmol (venous blood glucose > 10 mmol/l) is diagnostic, as too is a fasting venous plasma glucose ≥ 7.0 mmol/l (venous or capillary blood ≥ 6.1 mmol/l). In the absence of symptoms, these levels must be exceeded on two separate occasions. Impaired fasting glucose is a term used to describe individuals with raised fasting glucose not reaching the diabetic range. An oral glucose tolerance test should be considered in this group. This test also identifies a category of hyperglycaemia known as impaired glucose tolerance. This represents a stage at risk of progression to diabetes.

Classical symptoms include thirst, polydipsia and polyuria, weight loss, blurred vision and secondary infections such as thrush (oral, vaginal, balanitis) or skin infection. Many patients are asymptomatic at presentation, and the diagnosis may be picked up on incidental blood screening. Clinical assessment of elderly patients includes particularly measurement of weight, lying and standing blood pressure, peripheral pulses, examination of the feet for infection/ulceration, lower limb sensation, visual acuity and examination of the retina.

Management

The aim of treatment is to relieve symptoms, prevent acute metabolic complications and prevent long-term complications. Research has shown that improved care of diabetic patients can reduce both morbidity and mortality, although tight control of cardiovascular risk factors may have a greater effect than control of blood glucose concentration. This applies equally to old and to younger subjects. Improved glycaemic control is associated with reduced microvascular complications. Tight blood pressure control reduces both micro- and macrovascular complications. A National Service Framework for diabetes care has been introduced. Care is mainly provided in primary care with regular surveillance for long-term complications, with links established with secondary care for specialist involvement.

Tight diabetic control is usually the aim in preventing long-term complications, but this may not be appropriate for elderly patients who may be put at risk of hypoglycaemia, and, for elderly patients with limited life-expectancy, the long-term benefits of tight glycaemic control may not be achieved in their lifetime. The primary aim in this scenario is to control blood glucose to control hyperglycaemic symptoms and avoid hypoglycaemia. Interestingly, the type and severity of complications of diabetes may also be genetically determined: there is considerable variation in the type and severity of complications independent of the effectiveness of blood glucose control.

Patient education is central to diabetes care. Life-style modification includes review of diet, smoking and alcohol intake, promoting weight loss where appropriate and promoting exercise where feasible. Assessment of cardiovascular risk includes blood pressure (BP) measurement and lipid profile measurement. Urinalysis for microalbuminuria is performed regularly to detect early nephropathy. Progress to proteinuria and to uraemia may occur. Attention is required for the presence of foot problems related to neuropathy or vascular disease. Diabetic retinopathy screening is performed yearly.

Hypertension is common in diabetes, and a lower target BP of 130/85 mmHg has been suggested, although this may not be an appropriate target for elderly patients. Angiotensin converting enzyme inhibitors (ACEI) and angiotensin-2 receptor blockers (A_2 blockers) have advantages in diabetic renal disease, and should be considered for blood pressure control. Several drugs are often required to achieve BP control. They are also used if microalbuminuria develops, regardless of blood pressure. All patients with established vascular disease are prescribed statins to reduce cardiovascular risk. Cardiovascular risk is assessed to determine whether statins are used for primary prevention.

Symptom resolution indicates improved control clinically. Patients or their carers can monitor blood sugar using reagent strips and a glucose meter. Monitoring is essential for those patients on insulin. Frequency of monitoring will depend on disease stability and intercurrent illness. Patients may test themselves throughout a day, or check levels at different times on different days. The value of monitoring blood sugar in type 2 diabetes is less clear. Glycosylated haemoglobin (Hb_{AIC}) indicates blood sugar control over the preceding 1–3 months, and is used to monitor longer term control. Levels below 6% are normal. Guidelines suggest aiming for levels below 7%, but this degree of control may place elderly patients at undue risk of hypo-glycaemia. A target level of fasting glucose in venous plasma of < 5.5 mmol/l and 2-h postprandial level of < 7.8 mmol/l are too strict for the elderly, and < 7.8 mmol/l fasting and < 11.1 mmol/l 2-h postprandial levels are more appropriate.

Choice of treatment

For some older patients, reasonable diabetic control may be achieved through life-style and dietary modification alone. For those subjects in whom glycaemic control is not achieved, medication is required. Sulphonylureas and meglitinides increase insulin secretion from the pancreas. Biguanides decrease hepatic gluconeogenesis and enhance glucose uptake in muscle (and do not cause hypoglycaemia). Thiazolidinediones enhance insulin sensitivity in the liver, muscles and adipose tissue. α-Glucosidase inhibitors delay carbohydrate absorption. Patients with cognitive impairment may need medication supervision. Many elderly patients with diabetes treated with insulin require district-nurse care to manage their diabetes.

Metformin is the only currently available biguanide and is the drug of choice, especially in overweight/obese patients. It is contraindicated in heart failure, or renal or hepatic impairment. Gastrointestinal side-effects of nausea, diarrhoea and anorexia are common (25%).

Short-acting sulphonylureas such as glipizide are recommended in the elderly, as older, longer-acting preparations have a greater tendency to cause hypoglycaemia. They are used primarily in non-obese patients: they tend to cause weight gain. Thiazolidinediones are a new class of drug used alone or in combination with a sulphonylurea or metformin. As monotherapy they are not associated with hypoglycaemia, but may be ineffective if there is insufficient endogenous insulin. They can cause oedema and are contraindicated in heart failure and also in active liver disease.

Meglitinides are a new class of non-sulphonylurea secretagogue. Their role in the elderly is not yet clear, but they have an advantage in those who eat irregularly, as a tablet is taken immediately before eating; if a meal is to be skipped, a tablet is not taken. α-Glucosidase inhibitors target postprandial hyperglycaemia and do not produce hypoglycaemia. They may produce flatulence and diarrhoea, which limits their use.

Oral agents may fail to control blood glucose levels when used as monotherapy, and combination therapy may be required. Many patients ultimately require insulin therapy to achieve and maintain acceptable control.

Diabetic emergencies

Diabetic ketoacidosis (DKA) is a state of severe uncontrolled diabetes due to insulin deficiency characterised by hyperglycaemia, acidosis and ketosis. Although most diabetes in the elderly is non-insulin dependent, DKA can occur. The precipitant is usually infection. Symptoms can be non-specific such as general deterioration or confusion or include thirst and polyuria, weight loss, weakness, drowsiness and coma. Dehydration hypotension, tachycardia and hyperventilation may be seen. Bedside testing of blood glucose using a reagent strip and urine testing for ketones (Ketostix®) should be done. Suspected cases should be referred as an emergency to the medical team.

Hyperosmolar non-ketotic diabetic coma (HONK) is characterised by marked hyperglycaemia and dehydration without significant ketosis or acidosis. It is typically seen in elderly patients with type 2 diabetes, many of whom have not been diagnosed previously. Infection, diuretic therapy and the consumption of glucose-rich drinks can precipitate HONK. Symptoms may be similar to those in DKA. High blood glucose without ketonuria suggests HONK. Again, urgent medical referral is required.

In hypoglycaemia, symptoms are caused by autonomic activation (sweating, anxiety and palpitations) and neuroglycopaenia (confusion, drowsiness, tiredness, weakness, trembling, difficulty speaking, blurred vision and even epileptic seizures). It is seen in insulin-treated patients and in those on sulphonylureas. Hypoglycaemia occurs when there is a mismatch between the timing or dose of insulin/sulphonylurea and food. It is common with intensive treatment, and can occur with alcohol excess. Male gender, polypharmacy and increasing age are also recognised risk factors. Cognitively impaired elderly subjects may forget food or repeat medication and develop hypoglycaemia.

Any unwell patient with diabetes on insulin or sulphonylurea should have blood glucose measured. Any unconscious patient should have blood glucose measured by reagent strip testing at presentation. Immediate management consists of giving quick-acting carbohydrate orally as 25 g of glucose or 100 ml of sugary drinks (Lucozade®, or Coca Cola®) or jam, either eaten or smeared on the gums. Intravenous glucose, 50 ml of 50%, can be given. Glucagon, given subcutaneously or intramuscularly, can be used in type 1 or insulin-treated type 2 diabetes, but it should not be used for sulphonylurea-induced hypoglycaemia. Patients usually come around within minutes, and the next step is to avoid another episode. If the patient has had a significant hypoglycaemic episode and is on an intermediate/long-acting insulin or sulphonylurea, they should probably be observed for at least 24 hours with regular reagent strip monitoring, possibly with intravenous glucose infusion for 24 hours. Such patients should be referred for a medical opinion. Further management is aimed at determining the cause of the episode(s) and preventing recurrence.

Intercurrent illness means that diabetic patients may not be able to eat. For insulin-treated diabetes patients, this is a particular problem. In hospitalised patients, intravenous glucose and insulin may sustain the patient until oral intake can be resumed. Patients on sulphonylureas are also at risk of hypoglycaemia if oral food intake is inadequate. Management depends on the severity of the intercurrent illness and the patient's ability to eat and drink. Food supplements may sustain patients until a normal diet is resumed. Treatment for diabetes may need to be reduced in dose. If no intake is possible, intravenous glucose is almost always required. Such patients should be referred for medical advice.

Most hospitals have specialist nurses involved in diabetes care and offer liaison services. They are a good starting point for advice on diabetes care. Diabetic emergencies should be urgently referred to the medical team. Referral to the diabetic medical team may be appropriate for non-acute problems.

DIARRHOEA

The term diarrhoea usually refers to frequent or loose stools. However, some patients may actually mean faecal incontinence or faecal urgency: this needs to be clarified.

Diarrhoea of acute onset usually turns out to be infective or related to medication. In a hospital environment, particularly when cleaning protocols are inadequate and hand-washing by members of staff is not rigorously practiced, infective diarrhoea can spread rapidly and lead to ward closures. If there is an outbreak of infective diarrhoea, patients most at risk are those with gastric hypoacidity. Gastric hypoacidity is most often caused by previous gastric surgery, atrophic gastritis or the prescription of antacids or proton pump inhibitors.

Gastroenterologists view diarrhoea as the passage of more than 200 g of stool per day, or three or more watery stools in a 24-hour period.

Conventionally, acute diarrhoea has been present for less than 2 weeks. When diarrhoea has been present for more than 2 weeks and particularly for 4 or more weeks, it is referred to as chronic diarrhoea.

Four mechanisms underlie the development of diarrhoea:

(1) *Osmotic diarrhoea* This arises from the presence in the gut lumen of a substance that cannot be absorbed and which is osmotically active, leading to a net transfer of fluid into the lumen. Common causes of osmotic diarrhoea include a variety of laxatives and antacids containing magnesium salts, colchicine, cholestyramine and neomycin. Conditions resulting in malabsorption can also lead to osmotically active substances and osmotic diarrhoea.

(2) *Exudative diarrhoea* This commonly results from infection. It can also arise in coeliac disease, Crohn's disease, ulcerative colitis and a number of rarer conditions.

(3) *Secretory diarrhoea* This occurs because of mucosal stimulation of active chlorine ion transport. This mechanism is employed by some bacterial toxins and some rarer conditions.

(4) *Altered intestinal transit* This occurs, for example, in thyrotoxicosis.

Most cases of acute diarrhoea result from more than one pathophysiological mechanism.

Acute diarrhoea

In a service dealing largely with older people, ischaemic colitis should always be considered as a possible cause. Also, for in-patients especially, *Clostridium difficile* must be actively sought. Bloody diarrhoea or diarrhoea that is positive for blood on stick testing is very suggestive of inflammatory diarrhoea of colonic origin. Tenesmus may also be present. Voluminous and watery stools suggest disorders of the small bowel. Secretory diarrhoea persists despite fasting, and occurs both in the daytime and at night-time, in contrast to osmotic diarrhoea. If vomiting is a dominant symptom, this suggests 'food poisoning' caused by a toxin-producing bacterium or possibly a virus. The drug history always needs to be specifically addressed by both asking the patient and reviewing any prescription charts. It is important to make an assessment of the severity of the illness and whether the patient would be better managed on a medical ward.

Management

Most diarrhoeal illnesses are self-limiting and of mild to moderate severity. The stool should be tested for blood if no gross blood is present. It should also be sent for culture. Routine assessment for ova, cysts or parasites is generally unrewarding and is not recommended for routine practice. Exposure to antibiotics or acquisition of the diarrhoeal illness in hospital or some form of residential care should prompt a sample being sent for *C. difficile* toxin. The sensitivity of this test is about 85%, so more than one sample may need to be sent. For most patients, maintaining hydration is all that may be required. Suitable salt solutions are manufactured by several companies and include Dioralyte®, Electrolade® and Rehidrat®. During infective gastroenteritis, lactose intolerance may arise, and it is advised that milk and other lactose-containing products should not be given until recovery has taken place. Generally, it is not advised to give antimotility agents such as loperamide as they tend to prolong the illness and may even be harmful. If in doubt, seek advice.

Outbreak diarrhoea will usually be caused by a virus or *C. difficile*. The local 'Infection Control Committee' will usually supervise the management of the outbreak.

Chronic diarrhoea

Differentiating acute diarrhoea from chronic diarrhoea is arbitrary but practically useful, as the likely causes tend to differ as chronicity develops. For our purposes, chronic diarrhoea is that which has been present for more than 4 weeks. Probably the most important conditions to consider in the setting of an old age psychiatry service are laxative excess, other medications, thyrotoxicosis, faecal loading with bypassing and leakage of liquid stool and faecal incontinence. Most other causes require detailed investigation and an appropriate referral should be made. The likely causes are:

(1) Chronic watery diarrhoea:

   (a) Osmotic laxatives;

   (b) Other drugs (e.g. metformin);

   (c) Inflammatory bowel disease;

   (d) Cancer;

   (e) Diabetic autonomic neuropathy;

(f)   Vasculitis;

(g)   Hyperthyroidism;

(2)   Chronic inflammatory diarrhoea:

(a)   Inflammatory bowel disease;

(b)   Ischaemic colitis;

(c)   Radiation colitis;

(d)   Cancer;

(e)   Infections;

(3)   Chronic fatty diarrhoea:

(a)   Malabsorption;

(b)   Maldigestion.

Drugs commonly associated with diarrhoea

Many drugs are associated with diarrhoea. We list the commonest ones below:

(1)   Acetylcholinesterase inhibitors (donepezil, galantamine);

(2)   Antacids;

(3)   Antibiotics;

(4)   Antidepressants (SSRIs);

(5)   Anticonvulsants (lamotrigine, sodium valproate);

(6)   Antiplatelet drugs;

(7)   ACEIs;

(8)   Bisphosphonates;

(9)   Diabetes treatments (metformin, repaglinide, rosiglitazone, sulphonyl-ureas);

(10) Digoxin;

(11) Histamine-2 (H_2) receptor blockers;

(12) Laxatives;

(13) NSAIDs;

(14) Proton pump inhibitors.

FALLS

The causes of falls are many and various. It is common to be unable to identify some clear explanatory cause. It is impossible to understand the mechanisms of falls, and the various components of the physical examination that need to be performed in patients who present with falls, without having a basic understanding of the physiology of balance.

Physiology of balance

Balance is all about maintaining a dynamically stable posture during displacement and movement. It has three basic components:

(1)   Sensory input;

(2)   CNS-integrating mechanisms;

(3)   Motor responses.

The three dominant senses for these tasks are:

(1)   Vestibular (semicircular canals, otolith organs);

(2)   Visual (pursuit, optokinetic and saccadic systems);

(3)   Somatosensory (pressure and joint perception).

Vestibular system

The vestibular labyrinth is anatomically associated with the cochlea (which subserves hearing) in the petrous temporal bone. The components of the vestibular labyrinth are the semicircular canals, utricle and saccule. The labyrinth is fluid-filled and movements in the fluid are sensed by hair cells. The semicircular canals sense angular acceleration of the head, whereas the utricle and saccule sense linear acceleration and gravity. The three semicircular canals are at right angles to each other. The lateral canals on each side are coplanar. The anterior canal on one side is coplanar with the posterior canal on the other. Thus, for movement in any plane, at least two semicircular canals code the activity for the CNS responses. The signals from the semicircular canals cease once the head acceleration ceases. In contrast, the utricle (oriented vertically) and the saccule (oriented horizontally) have sustained signals during static head tilt with respect to gravity.

Vestibular input is integrated in the brainstem. The eighth cranial nerve carries vestibular signals to the medial and superior vestibular nuclei. The second-order neurons project ipsilaterally and contralaterally in the medial longitudinal fasciculus to the third, fourth and sixth cranial nerves to produce conjugate eye movements equal and opposite to the head movements: the vestibulo-ocular reflex (VOR). This is modulated by visual and proprioceptive cues through a second VOR pathway. Without the VOR, gaze would not be stabilised during high-velocity head movements (walking, riding in a car, etc.), and visual acuity would decline.

Most of the input from the saccule and utricle synapses in the medial and lateral vestibular nuclei, from whence second-order neurons project to the anterior horn cells of the spinal cord through the medial (cervical cord) and lateral (rest of cord) vestibulospinal tracts (vestibulospinal reflex, VSR). The purpose of this is to make postural adjustment with respect to gravity. The remainder of the input relays to the extraocular muscles to produce rotational and vertical ocular adjustment during head tilt.

Ascending pathways from the vestibular nuclei signal conscious awareness of body orientation. The midline cerebellum modulates the final muscular activity of the VOR and VSR, particularly in relation to visual and ocular cues.

Visual

Saccadic eye movements VOR stabilises gaze during head movements by maintaining fixation on a stable target. To change the object of fixation requires the saccadic system. Voluntary changes in the object of fixation are generated in the frontal lobe (frontal eye field), which projects to the oculomotor nuclei. Involuntary saccadic movements occur through vestibular and optokinetic stimulation and serve to return the eye to a neutral position. All saccadic movements are rapid, conjugate and accurate. Accuracy is controlled by the midline cerebellum and fastigial nuclei. Conjugate deviation and velocity are controlled by the frontal eye fields.

Smooth pursuit eye movements These conjugate movements track slowly moving targets with foveal vision. The pathway involves the retina, occipital cortex, accessory optic tract, superior colliculi and vestibular nuclei. The vestibular nuclei project to the oculomotor nuclei to generate the movements. Smooth pursuit declines with age, visual acuity, target speed, sedative medication, and cerebellar and cortical lesions.

Optokinetic eye movements These are similar to slow pursuit but rather than being driven by foveal vision, they are driven by full-field peripheral vision, and thus sense movement. The neural pathways involved are the same as for smooth pursuit.

Interactions All these systems are designed to bring and/or keep objects of interest centred on the fovea for maximal acuity. The VOR does this when the head is in motion and the object of interest is stable. The visual tracking systems (saccadic, pursuit, optokinetic) are used when the object of interest changes. When both the head and the visual field are moving, these systems require modulation by suppressing and enhancing individual components. With vestibular impairment, pursuit and optokinetic movements are used as partial compensation. The main mechanism of regulation emanates from the midline cerebellum, and lesions here cause a variety of impairments:

(1) Decreased fixation suppression;

(2) Impaired pursuit;

(3) Impaired optokinetic responses to target motion;

(4) Poor gaze stabilisation.

Symptoms of impaired vestibulo-ocular interaction Vestibular input at rest is symmetrical and no movement is sensed. With any head movement, input becomes asymmetrical and the movement is detected, and the eyes move in the opposite direction to maintain fixation. If the movement is sufficiently large, a saccadic movement resets gaze to a new target. This slow movement and rapid resetting is jerk nystagmus (fast phase towards the direction of motion). Damage to one labyrinth decreases the input from that side and the brain interprets the asymmetrical input as movement (vertigo), and the eye deviates towards the damaged side, followed by a rapid saccadic movement to restore fixation (nystagmus). Within days, central processing systems suppress the nystagmus and the vertigo subsides. Bilateral vestibular damage is usually not associated with nystagmus and vertigo. Instead, patients experience oscillopsia (bobbing of the visual field) with head movement because of the loss of the VOR and slippage of images across the retina. The slippage is reduced through compensation by smooth pursuit and optokinetic movements. However, this compensation fails with rapid head movements, when blurred vision and oscillopsia are experienced.

Somatosensory input

This is mainly through pressure receptors in the feet and stretch receptors in the anti-gravity muscles around the spine. This information is utilised in simple spinal reflexes (as used in the 'ankle strategy' during displacement) and polysynaptic, long-latency reflexes involving brainstem and cortical integration ('hip strategy', 'step strategy' during larger displacements).

Maintaining balance

Somatosensory inputs and visual cues are compared with vestibular cues to produce appropriate motor activity to keep the body centred over the base of support. The ankle strategy corrects for small perturbations, the hip strategy for larger ones and stepping to widen the base of support for the largest perturbations. With vestibular loss, greater reliance must be placed on somatosensory and visual mechanisms. These are less precise than vestibular cues, and the ankle strategy may be used inappropriately for larger displacements, with an increase in the risk of falling. In older people, it is common to have both visual and somatosensory impairments which, with vestibular impairment (e.g. presbystasis), leaves no reliable mechanism to maintain posture control, particularly on irregular or compliant surfaces with low levels of illumination.

Falls in older people

One-third of over-65s report a fall each year, as do over half of institutionalised elderly. The highest incidence of falls is in the very old and those with multiple impairments. In the over-75s, falls are the leading cause of death from injury. Soft tissue injury is reported in 20% of fallers and 5% sustain fractures. Fear of falling with consequential restrictive life-style and social isolation is reported in 25% of fallers.

Falls can occur owing to intrinsic or extrinsic (environmental) factors. Many risk factors for falls have been identified. Age-related physiological changes are of lesser importance compared with co-morbid factors, the most important factor for fall risk. Surveys suggest that over-65s have 3–4 chronic health conditions. The most frequent co-morbidities contributing to falls are cognitive impairment, visual impairment, arthritis, lower-limb weakness/dysfunction and use of drugs with psychotropic or vasoactive actions. Falling is one of the 'geriatric giants' (instability). Any acute illness may present as a fall. The presence of multiple risk factors increases the risk of falls.

Conditions associated with falls

(1)   Neurological disease: stroke, Parkinson's disease, visual impairment;

(2)   Musculoskeletal disease: mechanical dysfunction of joints, arthralgia;

(3)   Foot disorders: deformity, calluses, poorly fitting footwear;

(4)   Drugs: sedative medication, e.g. benzodiazepines; vasoactive medication, e.g. antihypertensives; drug toxicity, e.g. phenytoin;

(5)   Alcohol: either alcohol excess or a consequence of chronic abuse;

(6)   Seizure: a rare cause of falls in the elderly;

(7)   Syncope: loss of consciousness due to temporary impairment of cerebral perfusion with spontaneous recovery (see pages 97 and 133);

(8)   'Funny turns': dizziness, vertigo, presyncope (see page 97).

Approach to a patient who falls

A detailed history of the fall is required. What was the situation? Were there any preceding symptoms, e.g. prodrome of a faint, vertigo, oscillopsia or dizziness? Was there loss of consciousness? If possible, a witness account of the fall should be obtained. A history of previous falls suggests ongoing risk factors and that the patient is at risk of further falls.

Any acute illness may present as a fall, so examination should be thorough. Examination of a patient who has fallen should include a search for any injury. Check the pulse for any rhythm disturbance. Check the BP: is it low? If the patient reports dizziness on standing, this may suggest postural hypotension: check lying and standing BP. Listen for any heart murmurs. Assess vision. Check footwear and look for foot deformity. Assess cognitive function. Perform a neurological examination for evidence of focal weakness, balance or coordination disturbance. Remember to observe the patient's gait (page 112). Asking the patient to repeat any precipitating activity may identify the cause of a fall. A 'get-up-and-go' test may identify balance and motor deficits (page 18).

Investigations should be guided by the history and examination. FBC, urea and electrolytes and ECG are appropriate baseline investigations. Those with presumed syncope/blackouts should be referred medically for further advice, as should those with vertigo. Physiotherapy will help with strength and balance training and the provision of walking aids.

Most geriatrics services will have a falls clinic or falls assessment proto-col, often including dynamic cardiovascular testing. Assessment of fallers should include an environmental safety assessment to remove clutter, assess lighting, position of electric plugs, etc. If possible, any drugs known to con-tribute to fall risk should be reduced or eliminated. Interventions aimed at reducing injury from falls include prescription of calcium and vitamin D and bisphosphonates. The role of hip protectors is not yet clear.

In closing, we strongly urge that you do not use the term 'mechanical fall': it has no meaning. All falls are mechanical insofar as they arise from the net effect of the gravitational force that a person exerts on the earth and that which the earth exerts on the person: the earth always wins. What peo-ple usually mean or imply by this term is that no (remediable) cause for the fall(s) has been found. We favour the terms 'unexplained fall(s)' and 'multi-factorial fall(s)'.

FEVER AND INFECTION

Fever is a physiological response: it is not an arbitrarily specified change in the core temperature of the body. It is a driven, up-regulation of the core temperature by resetting of the hypothalamic thermostat: the actual tem-perature reached will depend on the temperature around which ther-moregulation usually took place. For most humans, this is around 37°C. However, some older people thermoregulate around a lower set-point. It is also important to note that the core body temperature is not static but fluc-tuates over the 24-hour cycle by about 0.8°C, with the trough occurring at night, during sleep. The amplitude of this circadian variation tends to be lower in older people, although cycle length does not change. Prostaglandins are important mediators of the fever response and drugs which inhibit their production (NSAIDs, aspirin, paracetamol) inhibit the development of fever. β-Adrenoreceptors are also involved in fever, and their blockade may inhibit the development of fever.

Small mammals drive up their core temperature mainly by heat genera-tion, and their metabolic rate increases markedly. Large mammals, such as humans, rely less on this mechanism and more on preventing heat loss. Thus, the earliest change in their fever response is vasoconstriction in the skin and the extremities: the surface temperature of the foot will therefore fall rapidly. The patient will feel cold, may request extra clothes or blankets and may shiver, although shivering is less prominent in some older people.

For the core temperature to rise, heat generation and conservation must exceed obligatory heat losses. In some older people whose fever response was initiated in a colder ambient temperature than is usual in hospital, core temperature may not rise until some hours after the hospital admission. A further complication is that body temperature is usually measured at sites of heat loss (mouth, axilla, forehead), and the recorded temperature may not be a faithful proxy for the core temperature. A tympanic infrared thermometer will be a better proxy provided that it is used correctly, with the sensor of the thermometer pointing towards the tympanic membrane. Sites where the skin is insulated (e.g. by a mattress) will tend to equilibrate with the core temperature, and infrared thermometry or simply feeling with a hand should give a reasonable estimate of the core temperature. This, taken together with evidence of peripheral vasoconstriction and feeling cold in a warm environment, should point to the presence of fever.

Causes of fever

Fever generally implies the presence of an inflammatory disorder, but it can also arise as an idiosyncratic reaction to drugs or be associated with underlying cancers, especially lymphomas. Occasionally, fever complicates non-infective CNS disorders (usually associated with haemorrhage). Thus, the causes of fever can be summarised as:

(1) Infection;

(2) Inflammation (rheumatic diseases, inflammatory bowel disease);

(3) Cancer (especially lymphomas and renal cell carcinoma);

(4) Drugs;

(5) CNS disorder.

Fever should always be assumed to indicate infection until proved otherwise. The drugs most often associated with fever are antibiotics. Thus, patients with infections treated with antibiotics whose fever does not remit with the treatment may be having the wrong treatment, or they may have developed a fever secondary to the antibiotic. They may also have developed antibiotic-associated colitis, so ask about diarrhoea. In your practice, urinary tract and respiratory infections will be the commonest to be encountered: search for evidence of these first. If there is no such evidence, think from the head down about the possible causes:

(1) Meningitis (headache, neck stiffness, photophobia);

(2)   Sinusitis (sinus tenderness);

(3)   Otitis (ear pain, reduced hearing);

(4)   Pharyngitis (sore throat, cervical lymph nodes);

(5)   Endocarditis (known heart valve disorder, recent dental procedure, urinary tract instrumentation, podiatry treatment);

(6)   Pneumonia (cough, sputum, chest pain, breathlessness);

(7)   Abdominal (pain, altered bowel habit, nausea, vomiting);

(8)   Urinary (dysuria, frequency, suprapubic pain, loin pain);

(9)   Pelvic (discharge);

(10)   Prostate (lower abdominal pain, tender prostate);

(11)   Peri-rectal/peri-anal abscess (pain, swelling, tenderness);

(12)   Skin (abscess, redness, swelling);

(13)   Joints (pain, warmth, swelling);

(14)   Bone (pain, arthroplasty, other orthopaedic surgery).

Examination

Perform a complete physical examination, including rectal examination, if the cause is not obvious. Pay particular attention to those parts suggested by features present from the above list. If there is a rash associated with the fever, the potential for serious (or life-threatening) infection is much higher: refer urgently for advice.

Investigations

Investigations should focus on your provisional diagnosis of the cause of the fever. If you do not have a potential cause after taking a history and undertaking an examination, you are dealing with a fever of unknown origin (FUO). The following investigations may help:

(1)   FBC (white cell count increased or decreased);

(2)   Urea and electrolytes;

(3)   Liver function tests (cholecystitis, cholangitis, liver abscess, hepatitis);

(4)   Amylase (pancreatitis);

(5)   Stick test urine (include nitrite, blood and protein);

(6)   Microbiological culture (sputum, urine, pus, etc.);

(7)   Blood cultures (three pairs of bottles with blood taken at different times);

(8)   Chest X-ray;

(9)   Abdominal X-ray (if abdominal pain or other abdominal features).

Fever in a traveller should suggest malaria: ask the haematology laboratory to examine a thick blood film. If you still cannot define a likely cause, you need to refer the patient for a medical opinion. The degree of urgency will depend on the condition of the patient.

Management

We have outlined the management of respiratory infections on page 232, and of urinary infections on page 141. Do not start blind antibiotic therapy unless you have no option: misuse of antibiotics is the major factor in the development of resistant organisms such as methicillin-resistant *Staphylococcus aureus* (MRSA). It is far better to send cultures to the laboratory before starting antibiotics. If the patient is not unwell, and you cannot make an educated guess at the likely organism, it is better to await the results of cultures. If you really have no idea of the cause of the problem or the patient is unwell, seek medical advice. The patient should have parenteral fluids to keep up with the increased insensible losses.

FITS, FAINTS, BLACKOUTS AND FUNNY TURNS

Many patients have great difficulty explaining the sensations they are experiencing, and they may also use words recognised to mean one thing by the doctor, when they mean another thing to the patient: always check what the patient means. It is also helpful to get a witness description of the episode. If the episodes are recurrent, and especially if there are bizarre features, a home video-recording can be very helpful. It is helpful to try to establish a number of features:

(1)   Have the attacks been witnessed by someone else?

(2)   Is balance usually normal or not?

(3)   Is the onset sudden or gradual?

(4)   Was the mental state altered before the episode?

(5)   Was there a fall?

(6)   Was consciousness lost?

(7)   What is the patient like during the episode?

(8)   Is there a sensation of movement?

(9)   Is there a vague sensation of disequilibrium?

(10) Is there a warning?

(11) Is recovery rapid or slow?

(12) Was there tongue biting?

(13) Was there any pallor or flushing?

(14) Was the patient stiff or floppy during the episode?

(15) Does anything provoke the episode (e.g. head or neck movements)?

(16) What drugs is the patient taking?

(17) Is alcohol abuse a possibility?

(18) Are there bizarre features?

If consciousness is lost, the episode is usually called a blackout. However, patients intoxicated with drugs or alcohol often use this term to mean a failure to register new episodic memories during the episode, rather than loss of consciousness. We discuss blackouts in detail below. The factors associated with falls have already been discussed in detail. Episodes that seem bizarre may be psychogenic in origin, but always consider that the cause is most likely to be epilepsy first: some partial seizures can be very bizarre.

Blackouts

Consciousness may be lost because of reduced brain blood-flow or because of seizure activity (epilepsy). The incidence of episodes of loss of consciousness increases starkly with advancing age from the sixth decade onwards.

For most patients who experience blackouts, the episodes are short-lived and are followed by spontaneous recovery. However, loss of consciousness can be a presenting feature of some extremely serious and immediately life-threatening conditions. Loss of consciousness that does not recover promptly is generally termed coma. Coma is more likely caused by a medical condition that a neurological one. Serious conditions can also induce loss of consciousness followed by recovery (at least temporarily).

Serious disorders that may induce loss of consciousness with (at least temporary) recovery include:

(1)   Myocardial infarction;

(2)   Pulmonary embolism;

(3)   Dissection of the thoracic aorta;

(4)   Major internal haemorrhage (ruptured aneurysm, ruptured varices, bleed from an ulcer, etc.).

The most important tool for illustrating the aetiology of episodes of loss of consciousness is a description by a witness. It is well documented that people may lose consciousness and yet they may have no awareness or recollection that this has happened at all. The witness should be asked to describe the events immediately before the episode of loss of consciousness, how the person appeared during the episode of loss of consciousness and the pattern of recovery and its time course. Premonitory symptoms and prolonged recovery with the patient not feeling their normal self for a lengthy period is highly suggestive of a seizure. In most cases, whilst unconscious, the patient will feel stiff, look cyanosed and often goes on to develop jerking movements. Patients whose loss of consciousness is caused by a cardiovascular condition generally appear pale and feel clammy. The presence of nausea, sweating or flushing, particularly if there is a situational trigger, is strongly suggestive of neurocardiogenic syncope. A lack of prodromal symptoms in a patient with underlying heart disease strongly suggests a dysrhythmia. However, it is now well established that dysrhythmias may arise during certain epileptic seizures.

It is important to discern what the patient was doing immediately before the episode and whether they were lying, sitting, standing or moving. Postural hypotension seldom arises while sitting and never when lying down.

Sleep is a physiological form of unconsciousness that may sometimes complicate a clinical setting. Indeed, one of us, whilst listening to a particularly boring representative of a pharmaceutical company, felt himself drifting off to sleep. The next recollection was a sharp pain in the middle of the chest as the pharmaceutical representative was trying to resuscitate the doctor.

Drop attacks

The term 'drop attack' is often used, usually without a clear definition. In fact, there is no generally agreed definition. For our purposes, we refer to sudden falls which occur without warning, either with or without loss of consciousness. The term is not a diagnosis, but a description of what happens. Studies of drop attacks are difficult to interpret owing to the lack of consistency in defining either the nature of the attack or the nature of the population from which the patient comes. Thus, in reading about drop attacks in different textbooks, the emphasis may be on CNS causes, vestibular causes, autonomic causes or vertebrobasilar insufficiency. Regardless, there always remain a large number of patients in whom no firm diagnosis of underlying disorder is possible: the older is the patient, the less likely is a firm diagnosis.

Many of the causes are discussed elsewhere in this section, or in the section on falls (page 89). The known causes of drop attacks are listed in Table 4.2.

Patients presenting with drop attacks require a detailed history, paying special attention to the events immediately before, during and after the attack. A witness description may be invaluable. Usually, home videos will be impossible to obtain owing to the brief and rapid nature of the episode. The physical examination focuses on potential neurological, cardiovascular and vestibular disorders. Atlanto-axial instability follows neck trauma but is also a feature of rheumatoid disease. The fall is usually precipitated by neck extension.

If, after your assessment, a possible cause is indicated, make the appropriate referral to a geriatrician, neurologist or cardiologist, according to your presumed cause. If you have no idea what the cause may be, refer to a geriatrician.

Vertebrobasilar ischaemia (vertebrobasilar insufficiency)

The two vertebral arteries arise from the subclavian arteries and merge to form the basilar artery at the pontomedullary junction, eventually giving off the posterior cerebral arteries. Major branches of the vertebrobasilar circulation are the posterior inferior cerebellar arteries, anterior inferior cerebellar arteries and superior cerebellar arteries. The clinical features of vertebrobasilar insufficiency are determined by the structures supplied by these

Table 4.2 Known causes of drop attacks

Syncope	*CNS*
Neurocardiogenic syncope (vasovagal, orthostatic)	Startle reactions
Carotid sinus syndrome	Orthostatic tremor
Postprandial hypotension	Cataplexy
Dysrhythmia (fast or slow)	Paroxysmal kinesigenic choreoathetosis
Left ventricle outflow obstruction	Posterior fossa mass (tumour, arachnoid cyst)
Myocardial disease (low cardiac output)	Frontal lobe tumours
Medications	Normal pressure hydrocephalus
Cough	Colloid cyst of the third ventricle
Micturition	Fourth ventricle ependymoma
Epilepsy	*Degenerative diseases (Alzheimer's, Parkinson's, PSP, MSA)*
Complex partial seizures (frontal, temporal)	Aqueduct stenosis
Tonic seizures	*Cervical spine*
Atonic seizures	Atlanto-axial instability
Absence seizures	Vertebrobasilar ischaemia
Transient ischaemic attacks	*Neuromuscular*
Bilateral anterior cerebral artery ischaemia	Myopathies
	Myaesthenia gravis
Vertebrobasilar ischaemia	Neuropathy
Subclavian steal syndrome	Myelopathy
Vestibular	*Idiopathic*
Menière's disease	
	Psychogenic

PSP, progressive supranuclear palsy; MSA, multiple system atrophy

arteries. Vertigo is usually the dominant symptom and is usually associated with nausea and vomiting. The entire episode usually lasts a few minutes. During the attack, ataxia prevents walking. There may also be tinnitus, facial droop, diplopia, headache and paraesthesiae in the limbs. If the patient is standing when the attack starts, falls are common. Usually, by the time the patient is examined, the physical signs will have resolved. Treatment is usually by treating any vascular risk factors present, although there is little evidence that these treatments have any effects on the attacks.

Fits/epilepsy

A seizure is a stereotyped episode of abrupt onset that may manifest as a disturbance of consciousness, behaviour, emotion, or motor, sensory or autonomic function. From the clinical presentation, it may be assumed to have arisen from an abnormal, self-limiting, paroxysmal or excessive discharge of a group of cerebral neurons. Epilepsy refers to the tendency to have recurrent, unprovoked seizures. The International Classification of Epileptic Seizures is complex, and a simpler scheme is more useful for our purposes:

(1) Generalised seizures:

   (a) Tonic;

   (b) Tonic–clonic;

   (c) Atonic;

   (d) Myoclonic;

   (e) Absence (typical/atypical);

(2) Partial seizures:

   (a) Simple;

   (b) Complex;

   (c) Secondary generalised.

The circumstances under which you may see older patients with epilepsy include:

(1) Epilepsy presents for the first time in old age in one of your patients;

(2) A patient with chronic epilepsy survives into old age;

(3) A patient with epilepsy has developed a psychiatric complication;

(4) An opinion is needed on diagnosing non-epileptic seizures.

It will be obvious which of these categories a patient falls into. When it presents for the first time in old age, epilepsy is generally related to clinically apparent or clinically silent cerebrovascular disease. The recurrence rate of seizures is high, and it is recommended that anticonvulsant treatment is appropriate for a single unprovoked seizure. The seizure types most frequently encountered in those presenting for the first time in old age are generalised tonic–clonic seizures and complex partial seizures. Other generalised seizure types may occur sometimes, and they may escape diagnosis owing to unfamiliarity. Those with chronic epilepsy surviving into old age may show any and all of the types of seizures listed above.

Tonic seizures

Tonic seizures are generally brief and involve stiffening of the limbs and trunk; a fall follows (often backwards) that frequently results in injury. Consciousness may be regained before the patient hits the floor.

Tonic–clonic seizures

This is what most people easily recognise as a seizure. Typically, loss of consciousness precedes the tonic phase (brief limb flexion followed by extension, often with a vocalisation). The clonic phase, with repetitive limb jerking, follows. The whole body may be involved and injuries are common. There may also be frothing at the mouth, tongue biting, cyanosis and evacuation of the bladder or bowels. Recovery may take several hours.

Atonic seizures

These are associated with a sudden loss of muscle tone and a fall, often resulting in injury. One description is that it is like all the bones being instantaneously removed from the body.

Absence seizures

Typical absence seizures occur only in children and are characterised by transient loss of awareness and sometimes of muscle tone, without loss of posture. The EEG findings are highly characteristic. Atypical absence seizures, which also mainly occur in children, are similar but less well defined and less abrupt, and consciousness may be clouded.

Myoclonic seizures

These are rare in geriatric practice. They are characterised by involuntary, brief jerks, often on or soon after waking. The arms are the most often affected, often symmetrically.

Partial seizures

These start focally, but they may secondarily generalise. The clinical features will depend on which part of the brain is primarily affected. Most arise in the temporal lobe (70%), but they also arise in the frontal lobe (20%), parietal lobe (5%) and occipital lobe (5%). Because they generalise, the features at the beginning of the seizure aid most in localisation (Table 4.3).

Table 4.3 Partial seizures

Temporal lobe seizures	Gestural automatisms
Amnesia	Autonomic features
Altered sense of time	
Anxiety/panic/anger	*Primary motor cortex seizures*
Epigastric aura ('butterflies in stomach')	Clonic jerks of thumb or big toe
	Face or hand twitching
Déjà vu/jamais vu	Jacksonian march
Depersonalisation/derealisation	Salivation
Gustatory/olfactory hallucinations	Speech arrest
Dysphoria/euphoria	
	Parietal lobe seizures
Frontal lobe seizures	Sensory aura
Acute onset	Feels limb is moving or absent
Amnesia	Vertigo
No aura	
Asymmetrical tonic posturing	*Occipital lobe seizures*
Agitation	Blindness
Eye/head deviation	Rapid eye blinking
Vocalisation/speech arrest	Eye deviation
Jerking progresses up limb (Jacksonian march)	Visual hallucinations
	Headache
Frontopolar seizures	*Central autonomic seizures*
Associated with falls	Sinus tachycardia
Clonic jerks of arms/legs	Cardiac arrhythmias
Head and eye deviation	Flushing
	Sweating
Orbitofrontal seizures	Hyperventilation
Olfactory aura	

Simple partial seizures involving headache may be misdiagnosed as migraine and those with focal features as transient ischaemic attacks (TIAs).

Management of epilepsy

Routine CT scanning and EEG are not recommended unless a brain tumour is suspected. The EEG can be most useful to differentiate focal (onset) seizures from primarily generalised ones. It is generally unhelpful in differentiating epilepsy from the other conditions we discuss here. If the diagnosis is unclear and epilepsy is a strong diagnostic possibility, refer to a neurologist or to the geriatrics service. Having a correct diagnosis of epilepsy is very important before starting anticonvulsant medications. Also before starting them, it is worthwhile withdrawing any epileptogenic drugs, where possible.

Numerous drugs are now available for the treatment of epilepsy. The choice of drug will depend on the type of seizure, although most new-onset seizures in the old are partial seizures with or without secondary generalisation. The older anticonvulsants are best avoided. Phenytoin is difficult to use owing to its unusual pharmacokinetics (shared with aspirin and alcohol). A reasonable first choice is sodium valproate or lamotrigine: these are non-sedating, have few interactions (except with other anticonvulsants, and especially with each other) and do not cause osteoporosis. Gabapentin is also remarkably free of side-effects, but seizure control is more erratic with this drug than with the others.

Start sodium valproate at 500 mg daily, which may be sufficient for many patients. The commonest maintenance dose is 1000–1500 mg per day. It can be given as a single dose or via a twice-daily dose schedule. Measuring plasma sodium valproate is rarely needed.

Alternatively, start lamotrigine at 25 mg per day and increase to 50 mg per day 2 weeks later. Increase to 100 mg per day in another 2 weeks. A dose of 100 mg per day may be sufficient to control seizures in older patients: most will be controlled within the dose range 200–400 mg per day. It may be given in a once- or twice-daily schedule. When introducing lamotrigine, watch for the development of a rash, which is an indication for tapering the dose and withdrawing the drug.

Particular care is needed when adding lamotrigine in a patient taking sodium valproate and vice versa. When adding lamotrigine to sodium valproate, start with 25 mg on alternate days and increase at 25-mg doses every 2 weeks. More than 150 mg per day is seldom needed. When adding sodium valproate to lamotrigine, the dose of lamotrigine should be halved before starting the sodium valproate at 500 mg daily. Do not increase the sodium valproate dose for another 2 weeks, at which time the lamotrigine dose may need to be reduced further (based on plasma levels) to avoid toxicity.

Unless you are very familiar with anticonvulsants, further treatment changes should only be undertaken by someone with a special interest in epilepsy.

Funny turns

There is considerable overlap between the causes of falls, funny turns and blackouts. If it is clear that consciousness was lost, consider them as blackouts and manage the patient accordingly. If it is clear that consciousness was not lost, or if there is doubt about whether it was or not, it is best to assess the patient as outlined below.

The language that patients often use to try to describe what has happened to them may be extremely confusing for the doctor. The most important thing is to try to clarify what the patient means. Generally, we try to assign the symptom to one of three groups:

(1)   Vertigo (vestibular);

(2)   Dysequilibrium (hyperventilation, multisensory impairment);

(3)   Presyncope.

Vertigo is defined as a subjective or objective illusion of motion, usually rotation. In other words, the patient either feels that he/she is moving or spinning when they obviously are not, or that they perceive themselves as stationary while objects move around them. Vertigo indicates a vestibular disorder, usually affecting the ear, but sometimes the brain. Details of the physiology of the vestibular system and its role in balance are discussed in the section on falls (page 89) *Dysequilibrium* is a vaguer sensation of unsteadiness, and generally indicates neuromuscular disorders, cerebellar disease and multiple sensory impairments. *Presyncope* is most often referred to as light-headedness or a sensation that the person is about to faint but does not do so.

Assessment

Unless the history gives a clear indication that the problem may be presyncope, the rest of the evaluation should focus on the nervous system and vestibular function. Those with presyncope should be evaluated as are those with syncope (pages 97 and 133). If the patient's description is not easily understood by you in physiological terms, you might wish to try to reproduce the symptom. Hyperventilation can be induced by getting the patient to take repeated deep breaths for 30 seconds. Hyperventilation is often associated with a primary anxiety disorder or secondary to falls, when patients develop exaggerated anxiety on changing position, moving or attempting to walk. Vertigo can be induced by rotational chair testing, first in one direction and then in the other, and stopping the spin abruptly after four rapid rotations. If this reproduces the patient's symptoms, proceed to a vestibular examination. Sometimes, getting the patient to perform a Valsalva manoeuvre can reproduce the symptoms.

History

Ask specifically about vertigo and oscillopsia (see page 89). Vertigo is not always experienced as spinning: it can also feel like falling or floating. Vaguer sensations are more likely to represent CNS causes or multisensory impairments. You should make specific inquiry about auditory symptoms (deafness, tinnitus) and visual problems. Acute changes in visual acuity (e.g. after cataract surgery, new glasses) can induce visual blurring and instability on head movement and walking: this improves with adaptation over time. Neurological symptoms should be sought, particularly affecting the legs (weakness, paraesthesiae).

Examination

The external ear needs to be examined by otoscopy (wax, infection, masses). Test hearing clinically and consider obtaining pure tone audiograms. Assess visual acuity, ideally using a visual acuity chart, both with and without corrective lenses. You can assess the VOR using a hand held chart by reading with the head still and shaking it back and forth. A loss of more than two lines indicates a VOR impairment. Examine eye movements looking for diplopia and nystagmus: note the characteristics of the nystagmus.

The patient requires a cardiovascular examination, including the blood pressure in both arms. The Valsalva manoeuvre, 'expiration against a closed glottis', may be done, at least to reproduce symptoms: it is ideally done with beat-to-beat BP and heart rate measurements. The patient may develop syncope through this mechanism during straining and coughing.

You should also do a screening neurological examination (page 18) and an evaluation of the cranial nerves from the seventh downwards. Also, assess gait (pages 18 and 112) and balance (page 18). You should also consider positional testing for benign positional vertigo (see below).

The Valsalva manoeuvre

Expiration against a closed glottis is hard to explain to the patient, and it is easiest for you to press on the anterior abdominal wall muscles and ask the patient to push against your hand with their abdomen. This raises intrathoracic pressure which, in turn, reduces venous return. It is conventional to continue for 10 seconds and then to release the pressure. The normal response is that, immediately on performing the strain, the blood pressure rises by an amount equal to the increase in intrathoracic pressure (usually > 25 mmHg). While the strain is maintained, the blood pressure falls and the heart rate increases because the raised intrathoracic pressure impedes venous return: ventricular volume decreases progressively. The decreased blood pressure and stroke volume cause sympathetic activation, which increases heart rate. When the strain is released, for the next few beats, the blood pressure falls (decreased flow from empty pulmonary vessels). The blood pressure then overshoots that recorded before the test because of the continued sympathetic activation (increases peripheral resistance), increased venous return and increased stroke volume. This increase in pressure induces bradycardia by activating carotid baroreceptors.

If the left ventricular ejection fraction (LVEF) is moderately impaired, there is no overshoot in BP since sympathetic activation was already high before the test owing to the underlying heart disease. With marked impairment of LVEF, there is a 'square wave' response in which the BP is sustained throughout the manoeuvre (excess blood in pulmonary circulation) and there is no overshoot on release.

Differential diagnosis of dizziness

The differential diagnosis of dizziness is wide but we describe only disorders encountered in older people here:

(1)   Benign paroxysmal vertigo;

(2)   Multiple sensory impairments;

(3)   Menière's disease;

(4)   Ototoxic drugs;

(5)   Perilymphatic fistula;

(6)   Acoustic neuroma;

(7)   Head injury (post-concussion, temporal bone fracture);

(8)   Acute labyrinthitis.

Benign paroxysmal positional vertigo

This is probably the commonest cause of vertigo you will encounter. It is characterised by brief episodes of vertigo precipitated by head movements. There is usually no precipitating cause for the condition. Often, a patient will develop vertigo when turning over in bed. It has several characteristics:

(1) It starts several seconds after assuming the provocative position;

(2) It intensifies and then resolves;

(3) It seldom lasts more than 30 seconds, even if the provocative position is maintained;

(4) The nystagmus is characteristically torsional towards the undermost ear;

(5) The nystagmus is characteristically associated with vertical up (posterior canal) or down (anterior canal) component;

(6) Repeating the provoking procedure may produce a lesser, or no, response.

It is most often tested for (in the vertical canal) by the Dix–Hallpike manoeuvre. In our experience, it can be very difficult to undertake the necessary movements in very old people with mobility difficulties. An easier way of testing for vertical canal benign paroxysmal positional vertigo (BPPV) is the Semont manoeuvre (side-lying test). Even so, you will probably need an assistant to help you do it.

The patient sits on the edge of the bed with the legs hanging down and the neck rotated 45° away from the side to be tested. Maintaining the head position, the patient then quickly lies down towards the side being tested (head will be looking upwards). After a delay of a few seconds, the patient may complain of vertigo and develop nystagmus. The patient is then moved *en bloc* with the head position maintained to lie on the other side (head will now be looking down). Again, ask about vertigo and watch for nystagmus. Repeat the test for the other side. Note that fixation can suppress the development of vertigo and nystagmus, which is why the test is often done with the patient wearing Frenzel goggles, if available. These contain lenses which blur the patient's vision and prevent fixation. However, they magnify (and illuminate) the eyes from the examiner's perspective, which makes it easier to see the vertigo.

Occasional patients have BPPV affecting the horizontal canal. This can be tested using the 'roll test'. The patient lies supine with the head slightly flexed. The head is turned 90° to one side and the eyes are observed for horizontal nystagmus. The test is then repeated, turning the head to the other side. As with the Semont manoeuvre, fixation may suppress the response: Frenzel goggles overcome this problem.

If nystagmus is observed without the initial latent period, suspect a posterior cranial fossa tumour and refer the patient for further evaluation: an MRI scan is most appropriate.

Multiple sensory impairments

This arises out of aging changes interacting with disease processes. It is usually associated with changes in proprioceptive and stretch receptor input, changes in the vestibular system, changes in the integrative mechanisms in the brainstem and cerebellum, impaired vision and altered control of corrective movements through long- and short-latency reflexes. In addition, it is not unusual to have secondary problems with anxiety. Patients will generally have impairments on gait and balance testing, which cannot be attributed to a single cause. Problems are often worst with low light levels and on compliant walking surfaces.

Menière's disease

Menière's disease tends to be overdiagnosed. Classically, there is increasing unilateral tinnitus, often preceded by a feeling of fullness in the affected ear. Eventually, the tinnitus gives way to a severe episode of vertigo, often preceded by a 'pop' in the affected ear. The vertigo can last for hours–days. Hearing is impaired. Over time, as the deafness worsens, attacks become less frequent. Eventually, deafness is severe and the vertigo ceases. ENT surgeons prescribe a number of treatments, none of which is very effective.

Ototoxic drugs

The vestibular apparatus and the vestibular nerve can be damaged by several commonly used drugs:

(1) Antibiotics (aminoglycosides, semi-synthetic penicillins, sulphonamides, chloramphenicol);

(2) Loop diuretics (furosemide, bumetanide);

(3) Aspirin;

(4) NSAIDs;

(5) Quinine;

(6) Phenytoin;

(7) Antihistamines.

Even with therapeutic drug monitoring, aminoglycosides cause damage to the auditory and vestibular systems: they should be used with caution in older people.

Perilymphatic fistula

This is an abnormal connection between the perilymphatic space and the middle ear. It can arise after surgery, ear or head trauma and barotrauma. Symptoms include hearing loss, tinnitus and episodic vertigo. It is usually managed by strict bed rest and vestibular sedatives, awaiting spontaneous closure. A failure to respond may be followed by surgery.

Acoustic neuroma

This is a benign tumour which produces its effects by nerve compression. Often, the first symptom is unilateral high-pitched tinnitus. True vertigo is rare, but the patient feels unsteady. As the tumour enlarges, there may be facial numbness and weakness. There is sometimes a headache.

Examination reveals sensineural hearing loss, lost corneal reflex on the affected side and facial sensory loss and/or weakness: the weakness is of the lower motor neuron type and affects the forehead too. There is decreased sensation in the external auditory meatus. Ipsilateral cerebellar signs may be present. If the tumour is large, there can be papilloedema. In patients with neurofibromatosis, there can be bilateral tumours.

Head injury (post-concussion, temporal bone fracture)

Post-concussional vertigo is generally severe, unilateral and positional. It tends to improve with time. Temporal bone fractures may damage either the middle ear (may be blood in the ear) or the labyrinth (also facial palsy). Both may cause vertigo and nystagmus. These patients should be referred to an ENT surgeon.

Acute labyrinthitis

This causes sudden onset of severe vertigo, exacerbated by head movements, and which subsides over several days. It is often associated with features of an upper respiratory infection (page 79). Sometimes, with influenza, recovery may take several weeks.

Management

Patients with hyperventilation associated with movement respond best to a structured physical rehabilitation programme with the input of an experienced physiotherapist and a clinical psychologist. Patients with clear vertigo are probably best assessed by an ENT surgeon, except that many geriatricians feel confident in performing repositioning manoeuvres when the diagnosis is clearly benign positional vertigo.

Even after a very detailed assessment, it is not unusual to have no precise diagnosis in around 30% of patients. Even when specific causes are identified, treatment is often unsatisfactory. For most patients the major outcome of concern is the prevention of falls and injury and the preservation of independence. Thus, the home environment needs to be assessed for hazards and the patient needs to be engaged in a falls prevention programme. This often comprises strength, conditioning and balance. Walking aids are provided as indicated. Visual impairments need to be corrected. Medications predisposing to falls need dose reduction or withdrawal of the drug. 'Vestibular sedatives' are generally not effective except in acute peripheral vestibular disorders: scopolamine patches may be the most appropriate treatment.

GAIT

Gait does not change greatly until age is advanced. Aging leads to a reduced walking speed and a wider stance. Stride length is shortened, with increased double support time (both feet on the ground at the same time) and reduced single support time. When assessing gait, pay special attention to knee, foot and ankle movements. In normal walking, the heel strikes the floor with the ankle dorsiflexed and the weight of the body is carried through the other foot. As the body moves forwards, the first foot flexes and then extends to take the body weight. Then the second foot flexes and pushes off against the floor. Arm movements reciprocate with the legs: as one foot comes forwards, so does the opposite arm. If the gait appears normal, test tandem walking (heel–toe walking), although many older people struggle with this.

Abnormal gaits are seen in a variety of disease states. A number of gait patterns are thought to be classical:

(1) Myopathic;

(2) Neuropathic;

(3) Spastic;

(4) Hemiplegic;

(5)   Ataxic;

(6)   Foot drop;

(7)   Extrapyramidal;

(8)   Subcortical;

(9)   Apraxic;

(10) Antalgic;

(11) Cautious;

(12) Psychogenic.

Myopathic

Proximal muscle weakness may lead to a waddling gait. Patients usually complain of difficulties climbing stairs and rising from chairs. There is an increased lumbar lordosis and the abdomen appear protruberant. This type of gait is seen with muscular dystrophies, proximal myopathies, myasthenia gravis and motor neuron disease.

Neuropathic

This is classically high-stepping. Examination reveals distal weakness and sensory loss with reduced reflexes.

Spastic

This is classically a scissor gait with bilateral leg weakness. The legs are stiff and steps are short. The knees are adducted and may cross during walking. There is little ankle movement. The toes may be dragged along the floor. The reflexes are usually exaggerated and there is a sensory level indicating the level of the spinal cord that is damaged. Bladder function is usually impaired. Patients with multiple sclerosis often have additional cerebellar involvement and there may be trembling as the foot makes contact with the floor.

Hemiplegic

The hemiplegic gait following a stroke typically leads to swinging out (circumduction) of the affected leg which is held in extension; the arm is held adducted at the shoulder, flexed at the elbow and wrist with the forearm pronated. Owing to modern rehabilitation practices to suppress spasticity, this sort of gait is seldom seen nowadays.

Ataxic

This is usually broad-based and staggering with irregular steps (length and frequency). There will be either limb ataxia with cerebellar hemisphere lesions or truncal ataxia with midline cerebellar lesions. With cerebellar hemisphere lesions, there will be nystagmus and the person will deviate towards the side of the affected hemisphere. Disorders of the frontal lobes may also produce a form of gait ataxia.

Sensory ataxia arises from dorsal column damage. It is usually broad-based, staggering and often high-stepping with slapping of the foot down on the floor, but with less lurching and reeling. Patients usually watch the floor where they are stepping. There is usually distal sensory loss but little by way of weakness. The problems are often much worse in the dark. This sort of gait may be seen in cervical myelopathy.

Foot drop

Foot drop usually leads to a high-stepping gait to avoid the toe hitting the floor. This is most often seen after damage to the peroneal nerve as it winds around the head of the fibula: sensory changes are usually absent.

Extrapyramidal

Parkinsonism

The gait is often the first thing affected in Parkinson's disease. Walking slows and is often cautious. The steps get shorter and shuffling then emerges. As the disease progresses, the knees and hips tend to flex. Later, the patient shuffles along, appearing to try to walk on the toes. The hands are often held near the thigh or lower abdomen, with little or no arm swing. Small obstacles may cause trips. There may be difficulties starting and stopping walking and there may be problems turning. By this stage, other features of the disease will have emerged in the form of tremor, rigidity and akinesia.

Dystonia

Dystonic gaits may occur in these patients as a result of treatment of the disease. Dystonic gaits are also seen with other forms of dystonia. There are abnormal leg postures, often induced by walking. Characteristically there is inversion and plantar flexion of the foot, and there may be toe-walking.

Progressive supranuclear palsy

Patients with progressive supranuclear palsy have a similar gait to that of Parkinsonism except that the neck is extended (retrocollis) and there is axial rigidity. The characteristic impairment of upwards gaze is frequent.

Chorea

Chorea affecting the legs causes bizarre lurching or stumbling in an irregular and unpredictable manner. This can be misdiagnosed as psychogenic.

Subcortical

The patient stands upright and there are short, small steps. There is usually a history of strokes. There may be pseudobulbar palsy and dementia.

Apraxic

This is usually slow in onset and gradually progressive. Early on, the patient walks with the feet close together and takes small steps: hips and knees are often flexed. There are frequent pauses followed by another series of steps. As the disorder progresses, initiating walking becomes more and more difficult, as if the feet are glued to the floor. When the patient is examined in a chair or on the bed, neurological signs may be minimal and the patient may be able to mimic walking movements. Dementia may be present and it may not. Not all demented patients develop gait apraxia.

Antalgic

An antalgic gait occurs with pain in leg joints. It may be limping, and sometimes staggering. There are usually no abnormal neurological signs. The Trendelenberg test may be positive.

Cautious

The patient walks with small steps and holds on to furniture. They usually express a fear of falling. This occurs after falls or with visual impairment and vestibular disorders.

Psychogenic

This is bizarrely staggering but without falls.

Further assessment

The patient requires a neurological and locomotor examination. There are no special tests that you need to order. Some specialist centres have facilities for computerised gait analysis. If you are confused, refer for help from a geriatrician or a neurologist.

GYNAECOLOGICAL PROBLEMS IN OLDER WOMEN

Gynaecological problems are not as common a health problem as in younger women. Postmenopausal changes include shrinkage of both the ovaries and the uterus. Vaginal atrophy owing to oestrogen lack is associated with thinning of the vaginal epithelium with reduced secretions of alkaline pH. There is vulval skin shrinkage with epithelial thinning. Aging also produces pelvic floor weakness.

Most gynaecological problems will probably require referral to the gynaecology team. Examination will require external inspection, bimanual examination and possibly speculum examination – these may best be left for the gynaecologist.

Clinical presentations include itching (pruritus vulvae), vaginal discharge, postmenopausal bleeding and urinary incontinence.

Vulval disorders

Vulval skin may be involved in generalised skin disorders or infestations, and is also subject to specific conditions. The most common symptom is pruritus vulvae, which may be due to infection, atrophic change itself, generalised skin disorder and specific vulval conditions. Lichen sclerosis is an atrophic process with plaques of keratin. Fusion of tissue may occur. Skin changes due to scratching may complicate the appearance. The condition can be premalignant and atypical areas should be biopsied. Lichen planus may also arise, and may appear like atrophic vaginitis unresponsive to oestrogens: it may occur simultaneously with oral lichen planus.

Squamous carcinoma of the vulva is seen most frequently in women in their 60s and 70s. Pruritus, or a lump, may be noticed by the patient. Late presentations include bleeding or discharge. Treatment is surgical. All suspicious vulval skin lesions should be referred.

Uterovaginal prolapse

This is usually seen in parous older women. Symptoms depend on severity and may include a bearing-down sensation, noticing 'a lump underneath' or urinary symptoms such as incontinence, urgency or a sensation of incomplete bladder emptying. Surgery is considered for more severe prolapse. Ring pessaries may be used in more minor prolapses or in those unfit for operation.

Vaginal discharge/postmenopausal bleeding

Most vaginal discharge is physiological. A change in usual vaginal discharge is an indication for further investigation. Causes include atrophic vaginitis, infection, tumours and foreign bodies. Blood-stained vaginal discharge should not be attributed to atrophic vaginitis without further assessment.

Endometrial carcinoma is the commonest malignancy of old age and usually presents with bleeding. Carcinoma of the cervix usually presents with bleeding or discharge.

HEADACHE

Although some conditions characteristically occur in older age, the incidence of headache declines overall. Cluster headache, cranial arteritis, trigeminal neuralgia, post-herpetic neuralgia and hypnic headache are all more common in old age. Headache may present as an acute problem or a chronic recurrent condition. As with most medical conditions the history will determine the diagnosis in the majority of cases. There are several important types of headache which will be considered in greater detail:

(1)   Headache associated with meningitis and subarachnoid haemorrhage;

(2)   Headache associated with temporal arteritis;

(3)   Raised intracranial pressure headache.

Patient assessment

Determine the anatomical location of the headache and whether it is unilateral, bilateral or shifting. Ask about the quality of the pain (constant, throbbing, sharp, dull, shooting, etc.). Is the pain worse at particular times of the day, month or year? Does the Valsalva manoeuvre (page 107) exacerbate the pain (suggesting raised intracranial pressure)? How severe is the pain? Does vision change in any way? Is there also jaw claudication? Finally, always look at the medication history.

Check pulse, BP and temperature. Are there signs of raised intracranial pressure (page 72)? Undertake a screening neurological examination looking for focal signs (page 18). Is there tenderness of the superficial temporal arteries. Spasm of the cervical muscles suggests greater occipital neuralgia: this may be associated with upper cervical tenderness and allodynia.

Acute new-onset headache

Serious underlying causes are much more likely in this setting. Conditions to be considered in this condition are subarachnoid haemorrhage, meningitis and subdural haematoma. Most patients are likely to need a CT brain scan urgently.

Worst-ever headache, abnormal neurological examination, fever, headache aggravated by coughing or lifting or headache present on waking suggest a serious underlying cause.

Raised intracranial pressure

This is bilateral, non-throbbing and worse in the morning. It may awaken the patient. The Vasalva manoeuvre (e.g. coughing, sneezing) makes it worse. There may also be vomiting. Focal neurological signs are usually present. The retina may show signs of raised intracranial pressure. If this is suspected, you are dealing with an urgent/emergency situation which may be amenable to treatment. An MRI scan and a neurosurgical consultation will be needed.

Meningitis

Patients with acute severe headache, neck stiffness and fever should be considered to have meningitis until proven otherwise. Patients should be referred medically for lumbar puncture.

Subarachnoid haemorrhage

Acute severe headache with neck stiffness without fever suggests this diagnosis. Patients with suspected subarachnoid haemorrhage (SAH) should be referred medically. A CT brain scan will usually demonstrate blood in the subarachnoid space. Lumbar puncture is often required to exclude SAH in the presence of a normal scan.

Temporal arteritis/giant cell arteritis/cranial arteritis

This is a condition of old age typically with inflammation of one or more branches of the carotid artery – characteristically the temporal artery branches. Headache is usually unilateral (but can be bilateral) and frontal. It is accompanied by scalp tenderness and tenderness over the affected vessels. Jaw claudication – pain on chewing food – may be present. Symptoms suggestive of polymyalgia rheumatica (pain and stiffness in the shoulder girdle) may also be present. Weight loss, anaemia and fever may occur as systemic manifestations. There is a risk of blindness due to involvement of the ophthalmic arteries. Suspected cases should be discussed urgently with the medical team. Patients usually have a high erythrocyte sedimentation rate (ESR) which must be checked. Ideally, the patient should be referred for temporal artery biopsy to confirm the diagnosis, but treatment with high-dose steroids should not be delayed especially if there are visual symptoms.

Recurrent headache

Tension-type headaches and migraine are the main causes of chronic recurrent headaches. Patients will usually give a long history of headache. Migraine may be accompanied by aura. New onset of migraine in old age is very rare.

Cluster headaches

This classically commences in older men as sudden-onset, severe, unilateral lancinating pain behind the orbit. It is often familial and may be precipitated by alcohol. The eye and nose may water on the affected side, and there may be a Horner's syndrome (ptosis and pupil constriction). The headache lasts 30 min to several hours and occurs in clusters, often with long periods without pain between the clusters. Acute attacks can often be aborted by inhaling 100% oxygen. Gabapentin may prevent episodes. Glucocorticoids and lithium may also be effective.

Tension-type headaches

These are bilateral, non-throbbing, constant headaches, usually spreading from the occiput to the frontal area, which are usually worse in the evenings. The pain may be described as squeezing or severe pressure. It is unaffected by the Valsalva manoeuvre. Allodynia may be present. Apart from spasm of the cervical muscles, the neurological examination will be normal. The pain is often severe at times of 'stress'.

Treatment is with simple analgesics, which are variably effective. Local heat and massage to the back of the neck may help. Other treatments which may help include cervical traction, gabapentin and local glucocorticoid injections.

Hypnic headache

This is a rare headache that appears to arise during REM sleep. It occurs more commonly in women. The headaches begin abruptly and are diffusely throbbing. They subside within a few hours. It is important to exclude raised intracranial pressure, cranial arteritis and cluster headaches. Treatment with lithium is said to be effective.

Exploding-head syndrome

This arises as a 'bang', 'clap' or 'explosion' in the head during stage 1 sleep. Pain is an inconsistent feature. There is no specific treatment: reassurance should be given.

Trigeminal neuralgia (tic douloureux)

This is a recurrent, paroxysmal pain in the distribution of one or more divisions of the trigeminal nerve. The pain may radiate to the jaw or teeth and present as a dental problem. The pain is often induced by even light touching of a localised area of the face. There is never any associated sensory loss or loss of the corneal reflex: if present, it should prompt investigation for neoplastic or vascular disorders involving the trigeminal nerve. The first-line treatment is gabapentin (page 241) and an antidepressant may be added. Patients who respond poorly to treatment should be referred to a neurologist or to a pain specialist.

Post-herpetic neuralgia

This follows an episode of shingles (zoster). There will often be residual scarring in the affected area. Management of shingles and post-herpetic neuralgia is discussed on page 150.

Medication headache

Many drugs are associated with headaches. Common ones include:

(1)   Nitrates;

(2)   Lithium;

(3)   Ephedrine;

(4)   Digitalis;

(5)   Tricyclic antidepressants.

Particularly in the setting of migraine or tension-type headaches, drugs, once effective, can exacerbate or maintain headache. Patients often take further medication, only to be followed by further headache, often more severe, thus causing a vicious cycle. Withdrawal of medications is often very difficult in such patients.

Temporomandibular neuralgia

This is usually severe, unilateral aching around the temporomandibular joint (TMJ). It may radiate to the jaw and the TMJ may be tender. The pain is exacerbated by lower jaw movements such as chewing and yawning. There may be nocturnal bruxism. In older patients, it is most often associated with overbite associated with the loss of molars. Treatment of the dental malocclusion may relieve the pain. Otherwise, treat with simple analgesics and a soft diet to limit mouth opening. If the treatment proves unsatisfactory, get the opinion of a maxillofacial surgeon.

HEAD INJURY

Head injuries vary considerably in type and severity and have diverse consequences. Approaching 10% of adults have a history of at least one head injury severe enough to cause loss of consciousness or confusion. Fall-related head injury is by far the commonest mechanism in the elderly. The sequelae relate to both direct effects (compression/contusion, diffuse axonal injury) and indirect (brain swelling, haematomas). The brain is not uniformly vulnerable to damage – the anterior surfaces of the frontal and temporal lobes are the most sensitive to deceleration forces, whereas the occipital lobe is most likely to be damaged during a direct impact (falling backwards). Shearing injury from rotational forces occurs in the white matter of the cortical, subcortical and limbic areas. A minority of such injuries are suspected clinically, although they can be demonstrated using special staining techniques at autopsy.

Head-injury severity can be defined in terms of the duration of unconsciousness (if any), Glasgow Coma Scale score and the duration of post-traumatic anterograde amnesia (and other immediate mental changes). Significant morbidity may arise in survivors of even mild head injuries (disorientation lasts < 15 min; no loss of consciousness; post-traumatic amnesia < 24 h). Epilepsy, permanent cognitive impairment, depression, psychosis, frontal lobe signs (frontal disconnection syndrome) and personality changes all occur more commonly than in the non-head-injured population.

Management of the head-injured patient

Loss of consciousness at the time of the injury is an indication to transfer the patient to an acute-care service, whereas the alert patient can be managed on the ward. Prior to transferring an unconscious patient, insert an oropharyngeal airway and apply suction to remove secretions. Perform a brief neurological examination looking for weakness/paralysis, tendon reflex changes and plantar responses. Assess pulse, blood pressure, pupil size and responses and Glasgow Coma Score every 15 minutes. Note any abnormal postures (see page 72). If there is any possibility of neck injury, take care not to move the neck and try to stabilise it – the ambulance staff will have the equipment to do this if you do not. Insert a cannula in case it may be needed in an emergency, but avoid infusing fluids unless the patient is hypotensive. Any seizures should be treated with intravenous diazepam (0.37 mg/kg up to a maximum of 10 mg), but otherwise, avoid giving any sedating drugs.

If consciousness is unimpaired and neck injury has not occurred, emergency transfer elsewhere is not warranted. However, the patient needs to be assessed for bruising, lacerations and scalp avulsions. If suturing is needed, this is best done in the A&E department. The patient requires measurement of pulse and blood pressure, pupil examination and a brief neurological examination, as described above. Record the Glasgow Coma Scale score every 15 minutes for an hour and then hourly thereafter for 24 hours.

If any new focal neurological signs develop, the patient should move to the acute-care service and a CT scan of the brain will be needed. Bruising over the mastoid (Battle's sign) suggests a basilar skull fracture. Bruising around the eyes (looking like a panda) suggests frontal bone fracture. These signs indicate the need for skull radiographs and transfer to the acute medical service. Otherwise, routine skull radiographs are not warranted. The development of focal neurological signs suggestive of internal herniations of the brain (see page 72) indicates that urgent transfer to a neurosurgery service is needed. If the patient remains well after 24 hours, the regular observations can safely stop. Recall the possible consequences of even mild head injuries listed above.

HEART FAILURE

Heart failure is mainly a disease of old age. It has a high mortality and morbidity. The patient's condition can fluctuate and deterioration can lead to hospital admission. The most common causes of heart failure are ischaemic heart disease, hypertension and valvular heart disease. Heart failure has a complex pathogenesis but occurs when the heart pump function is unable to meet the physiological demands upon it. Good evidence exists for improvement in mortality and morbidity with medical therapy. Symptomatic heart failure has a worse 1-year mortality than many cancers. Most heart failure is due to left ventricular dysfunction. In older patients, heart failure is frequently seen with normal left ventricular function but with abnormal diastolic filling and ventricular relaxation. This is known as diastolic heart failure.

The principal symptoms are breathlessness with exercise limitation and fluid retention. Patients may report orthopnoea – breathlessness when lying flat when heart failure is severe. Paroxysmal nocturnal dyspnoea is an acute episode of breathlessness at night, and is seen particularly in acute left ventricular failure. Patients may notice ankle swelling and weight gain. Elderly patients may present quite late because patients may not notice symptoms due to their limited exercise capacity. Examination may reveal ankle oedema or sacral oedema if the patient has been bed-ridden. The jugular venous pressure (JVP) may be raised. The apex beat may be displaced. An added third heart sound may be heard, and bibasal fine inspiratory crackles may be heard on chest auscultation. Hepatomegaly may be seen due to hepatic congestion.

Obesity and chest disease, severe anaemia and thyroid disease may present with similar symptoms. Oedema may occur with hypoalbuminaemia, renal and liver disease, chronic venous insufficiency, lymphatic insufficiency and as drug side-effects (e.g. calcium antagonists, NSAIDs). Gravitational oedema is common in immobile elderly patients and presents a diagnostic difficulty.

Symptoms, exercise tolerance and any functional limitation should be determined. Examination should include pulse rate and rhythm, BP measurement, assessment of JVP, auscultation for heart murmurs and added heart sounds, chest auscultation for basal crackles and assessment of ankle and sacral oedema. Abdominal examination should be performed for hepatomegaly.

Investigations of heart failure should include chest radiograph, 12-lead ECG, blood count, urea and electrolytes, liver function, thyroid function, glucose, lipids (as part of cardiovascular risk assessment) and urinalysis for protein. Echocardiography should be used to confirm cardiac dysfunction.

Management

The aim of treatment is to alleviate symptoms and to improve mortality.

Exercise is beneficial and is encouraged if feasible. Dietary salt restriction is advised. It is recommended that smoking is stopped, and alcohol intake should be limited. Excess fluid intake should be avoided (1.5–2.5 litres in 24 h recommended). Most patients will require drug therapy.

The use of drugs will be determined by tolerability and the presence of co-morbidity. ACEIs may be contraindicated in renal impairment, and beta-blockers may be contraindicated in COPD or asthma. Diuretics may precipitate gout and incontinence. Diuretics and ACEIs can lead to renal failure. Hypotension as a drug side-effect may lead to falls. The following classes of drugs are used commonly in heart failure.

Diuretics

Loop diuretics such as furosemide or bumetanide are used to relieve congestive symptoms and fluid retention. Doses may be titrated up or down as needed. Thiazide diuretics such as bendroflumethazide or metolazone are sometimes added in resistant heart failure. Spironolactone, an aldosterone antagonist, is added in more severe heart failure.

ACEIs

All patients with heart failure secondary to left ventricular dysfunction should be considered for treatment. Patients with valvular heart disease should have specialist assessment prior to commencing ACEIs.

Beta-blockers

These are added to treatment after diuretics and ACEIs. Careful titration is required. Carvedilol and bisoprolol are currently licensed in the UK. Elderly patients may not be able to tolerate beta-blockers for heart failure.

Digoxin

This may be added for patients with worsening heart failure already on the above drugs, and is also used in patients with atrial fibrillation and heart failure.

Angiotensin II receptor antagonists

Although not currently licensed for heart failure, they are sometimes used as an alternative in patients who are intolerant of ACEIs.

Monitoring

All patients require regular monitoring. The frequency will depend on the clinical status, stability and co-morbidity of each patient. Six-monthly intervals are reasonable for stable patients, more frequently if clinically indicated or if treatment is altered. Symptoms and functional status should be assessed with monitoring of weight, clinical examination and urea and electrolytes testing as a minimum.

Deterioration in symptoms can occur with uncontrolled hypertension, the development of atrial fibrillation, non-compliance with medication, myocardial ischaemia, anaemia, renal insufficiency, use of non-steroidal anti-inflammatory drugs and overindulgence in salty food.

Does this elderly lady patient with swollen ankles have heart failure?

Does she have symptoms? If not, heart failure is less likely. Could anaemia or thyrotoxicosis explain the symptoms (clinical examination plus blood tests)? Does the patient have a history of chronic lung disease?

Does she have any predisposition? A history of rheumatic fever (valvular heart disease), ischaemic heart disease or hypertension will increase the likelihood.

Could the ankle oedema be due to other causes? If the patient has been immobile then the oedema may be gravitational. Drugs such as calcium antagonists can produce oedema. Malnourishment (low albumin), chronic liver disease (history of alcohol excess, jaundice and abnormal liver function) and renal disease (urea and electrolytes plus urinalysis for protein) may also cause oedema. Weight gain suggests fluid retention.

Are there clinical signs of heart failure? The most useful signs are unfortunately the more difficult to elicit. Raised jugular venous pressure (JVP), a displaced apex beat and the presence of a third heart sound support the diagnosis.

Can investigations help? Yes. In 90% of patients an ECG will show some abnormality. Chest radiograph (CXR) may show cardiac enlargement or pulmonary oedema. A normal ECG and CXR have a high (but not perfect) negative predictive value. Echocardiography is the gold-standard investigation. Natriuretic peptides (B-type, BNP; and N-BNP, N-terminal BNP) are raised in heart failure. Their measurement is being considered as a way to screen suspected heart-failure patients for echocardiography. They may become more widely used in diagnosis, but their role in clinical practice is still being evaluated.

Common problems in patients with heart failure

The patient is hypotensive If the patient is asymptomatic, i.e. no light-headedness or fatigue and urea and electrolytes are unchanged, continue current treatment. In symptomatic patients, reduce the dose of diuretic initially.

The patient is hyperkalaemic Ensure that the patient is not taking any exogenous potassium, e.g. salt substitutes.

Consider decreasing the dose of potassium-sparing diuretic. Avoid high-dose ACEIs if the patient is on spironolactone. Avoid spironolactone if the patient is in renal failure.

If potassium is greater than 5.9 mmol/l, contact the medical team.

The patient's urea is climbing Decrease the dose of diuretic. Contact the 'on an ACEI' medical team for advice.

Getting help

The management of heart failure is becoming increasingly complex, and specialist help is often required. Acute deterioration will usually mean that the patient will require transfer to a medical/cardiology bed. The on-call medical team should be contacted. Patients may be referred to cardiologists or geriatricians for advice. Many patients with heart failure are now followed-up in nurse-led heart-failure clinics, and these specialist practitioners are another source of advice.

HICCUPS (SINGULTUS)

Hiccups are inspiratory sounds caused by abrupt closure of the glottis during reflex spasms of the diaphragm and muscles of ventilation. They are much commoner in men than in women and usually last only for a few minutes, although they occasionally persist for years.

Causes of hiccups

Hiccups have many causes, but all involve vagal stimulation, brainstem disorders or phrenic nerve activation. Gastric distension is the commonest cause, especially if there has been ingestion of a cold, fizzy drink. Other causes include:

(1)   Surgery (neck, thorax, abdomen);

(2)   CNS disorder (stroke, multiple sclerosis, brain tumour);

(3)   Electrolyte disorders (hyponatraemia, hypokalaemia, hypocalcaemia);

(4)   Uraemia;

(5)   Infection (lower-lobe pneumonia, subphrenic abscess, peritonitis);

(6)   Carcinoma of the pancreas;

(7)   Drugs (benzodiazepines, alcohol).

Treatment of hiccups

Most episodes subside without treatment. Many folk-remedies have been suggested which are probably not very effective. These include eating a teaspoon of granulated sugar, tongue traction, massaging the soft palate, drinking ice-water and a sudden 'scare'.

If these fail and the episode does not resolve spontaneously, metclopramide may be effective.

HYPERTENSION

Aging imposes several changes on the cardiovascular system which may, depending on circumstances, achieve practical relevance. First, large and medium-sized arteries lose elastin fibres and collagen is deposited. This increases the afterload and induces a modest increase in systolic blood pressure. Some older people have very marked increases in arterial stiffness and may deposit calcium in vessel walls. There is compensatory hypertrophy of cardiac myocytes. At the same time, there are changes in storage and transport of calcium (critical for muscle depolarisation), which leads to impaired relaxation of the ventricles in diastole and decreased ventricular compliance. Peak ventricular filling during diastole is late, which explains why older people tolerate rapid heart rates poorly. Nevertheless, owing to age-related changes in β-adrenergic receptors and responsiveness to agonists, older people become more dependent on preload to increase cardiac output in response to demand. Finally, there are degenerative changes in the conducting system from the sinus node downwards, which predisposes older people to both brady- and tachydysrhythmias.

Hypertension is common in old age. Advancing age is associated with a rising systolic blood pressure and relatively lower diastolic blood pressure. Isolated systolic hypertension is seen much more commonly. Treating hypertension is associated with a reduction in stroke, myocardial infarction and death. Increasingly, thresholds for treatment are falling, and more aggressive management is being promoted. In the elderly we know that treatment up to the age of 80 years is worthwhile. There are as yet no trial data to guide beyond that age, but studies are in progress. There are some epidemiological data relating high blood pressure to survival in octogenarians and nonagenarians. In practice, those already on treatment before 80 years of age carry on taking it once they reach 80 years, and patients over 80 years with evidence of end-organ damage are treated. Meanwhile, low target BP measurements are encouraged. The gain with this approach in elderly patients is not known.

Aetiology

Most patients will have primary or essential hypertension for which there is no underlying cause.

Secondary hypertension is much less common. Causes include chronic renal disease, renal artery stenosis, phaeochromocytoma, Conn's syndrome,

Cushing's disease, coarctation of the aorta and drugs including NSAIDS, liquorice, steroids and sympathomimetics.

Secondary hypertension should be suspected in the following circumstances. Hypokalaemia with normal or increased sodium might indicate Conn's syndrome. Elevated serum creatinine or proteinuria or haematuria might suggest chronic renal disease. Sudden onset or worsening of hypertension or resistance to a multidrug regimen, i.e. ≥3 drugs, should raise the suspicion of secondary hypertension.

Management

Clinical assessment

The aim of clinical assessment is to confirm the diagnosis, identify evidence of end-organ damage due to hypertension, detect conditions leading to secondary hypertension, assess cardiovascular risk factors and assess for possible contraindications to specific drug treatment.

Cardiovascular examination and fundoscopy for hypertensive retinal changes are essential. Routine investigations would include full blood count, urea and electrolytes, blood glucose and lipids (ideally fasting samples) and an ECG to look for evidence of left ventricular hypertrophy or evidence of ischaemic heart disease. Latest guidelines (Table 4.4) do not recommend routine urinalysis, chest X-ray or echocardiography.

Table 4.4 British Hypertension Society Guidelines: complications of hypertension/target organ damage

Stroke, TIA, dementia, carotid bruits   LVH and/or LV strain on ECG, heart failure
Myocardial infarction, angina, CABG or angioplasty   Peripheral vascular disease
Fundal haemorrhages or exudates, papilloedema   Proteinuria   Renal impairment (raised serum creatinine)

TIA, transient ischaemic attack; LVH, left ventricular hypertrophy; LV, left ventricle; ECG, electrocardiography; CABG, coronary artery bypass graft

Who do you treat?

There are various guidelines indicating treatment thresholds, targets and the selection of drugs. However, it is important to remember that you are treating a patient and not just a measurement.

The latest British Hypertension Society Guidelines (2004) recommend that treatment should be started in people with a sustained systolic BP (SBP) of ≥ 160 mmHg or sustained diastolic BP (DBP) of ≥ 100 mmHg.

The following thresholds for intervention are recommended:

(1)   If BP is greater than or equal to 220/120 mmHg treat immediately;

(2)   If BP is greater than 180–219/110–119 mmHg confirm over 1–2 weeks then treat;

(3)   If BP is 160–179/110–109 mmHg:

    (a)   If there are cardiovascular complications or target-organ damage or diabetes mellitus, confirm over 3–4 weeks then treat;

    (b)   If there are no cardiovascular complications, target-organ damage or diabetes mellitus, life-style measures should be advised. Measure BP weekly and treat if BP persists over 4–12 weeks;

(4)   If BP is 140–159/90–99 mmHg.

    (a)   If there are cardiovascular complications or target-organ damage or diabetes mellitus, confirm within 12 weeks, then treat;

    (b)   If there are a no cardiovascular complications or target organ damage or diabetes mellitus, life-style measures are advised and blood pressure should be re-measured at monthly intervals;

    (c)   If mild hypertension persists, estimate 10-year cardiovascular disease (CVD) risk formally, and if it is over 20% then treat.

Statin therapy is recommended for all hypertensive patients with CVD irrespective of baseline cholesterol, and for primary prevention in those over 40 years with a 10-year risk ≥ 20%. For primary prevention, this treatment, recommended for those up to 80 years, would mean treating most hypertensives over 50 years of age, and has considerable resource implications.

Low-dose aspirin is recommended for secondary prevention of CVD and for primary prevention in those over 50 years with a 10-year CVD risk of ≥ 20% and whose BP is controlled to < 150/90 mmHg.

The new General Medical Services (GMS) Contract for primary care will direct a major focus on the quality of care provided, with incentives and rewards for good practice. Hypertension assessment and treatment is covered in the contract, which should ensure that more hypertensive patients are targeted and treated.

How low do you go?

Whilst evidence for target blood pressure control is incomplete, generally, 'the lower the better' is believed to be the best approach. Even if the therapeutic target is not reached, there are still benefits to lowering blood pressure. On starting treatment, it is important to remember that aging imposes on the individual an altered body in which the drugs need to work. Aging changes and co-morbidity will tend to alter both pharmacokinetic and pharmacodynamic parameters, and care is needed to avoid adverse drug reactions.

In non-diabetics, the target BPs are SBP < 140 mmHg and DBP < 85 mmHg.

In people with diabetes, chronic renal failure or established CVD optimal BP goals are lower, at SBP < 130 mmHg and DBP < 80 mmHg.

Treatment options

Non-drug treatment: life-style advice

Life-style advice should be given to all patients. Advice addresses interventions both to reduce blood pressure and to reduce cardiovascular disease risk.

Interventions to lower blood pressure include: weight reduction, altering the diet to reduce fats, increase fruit and vegetables and restrict dietary salt (< 6 g NaCl), and promotion of exercise and moderate alcohol intake (men ≤ 21 units per week, women ≤ 14 units per week).

Stopping smoking, reducing fat and increasing unsaturated fat and increasing oily fish consumption reduce cardiovascular disease risk.

Drug treatment

The ABCD rule This is a guide to initiate drug treatment:

A   ACEIs, angiotensin receptor blockers;

B   beta-blockers;

C   calcium antagonists;

D   diuretics.

Younger patients tend to have high plasma renin: start treatment with A or B. Older patients (> 55 years) and black patients tend to have low plasma renin: start with C or D.

For older patients, if BP is not controlled try C or D + A or B; if BP is *still* not controlled try C or D + A and B. The combination of A + B + C + D can be tried but there is not a strong evidence base for this approach. Alternatively, add either an alpha-blocker or spironolactone or another diuretic.

Most patients will need two or more drugs to achieve control.

It is recommended to avoid B + D in those at risk of diabetes mellitus, i.e. strong family history, obesity, South Asian or Afro-Caribbean patients and those with impaired glucose tolerance. Future guidelines may look at the place of beta-blockers in treatment regimens, as they appear to potentiate the risk of diabetes mellitus.

Drug use will depend on the patient's tolerance and co-morbidity. For example, beta-blockers would be avoided in asthmatics, and thiazide diuretics might be avoided in gout or incontinence. ACEIs have advantages in heart failure, as do beta-blockers in angina.

Malignant or accelerated hypertension

This syndrome of very high BP, retinal haemorrhages and exudates with or without papilloedema is increasingly rare in UK practice. Patients may be asymptomatic. Headache and visual disturbance are the commonest symptoms. Breathlessness secondary to left ventricular failure may occur. Fluctuating neurological signs, disorientation, reduced consciousness, neurological deficit and seizures may indicate hypertensive encephalopathy.

Oral treatment is recommended unless there is gross heart failure, aortic dissection or hypertensive encephalopathy, when parenteral therapy is usually required.

Getting help

Patients with accelerated hypertension should be referred urgently to the medical team. Severe hypertension should also be referred urgently (> 220/120 mmHg).

If secondary hypertension is suspected, refer medically for further investigation. Patients with evidence of target-organ damage should also be referred.

HYPOTENSION

Recumbent hypotension is usually defined as a blood pressure of less than 90 mmHg. There is no agreed criterion for the diagnosis of postural hypotension, but it is commonly defined as a fall in systolic blood pressure of 20 mmHg or 10 mmHg diastolic blood pressure on standing or after 3 minutes of head-up tilt. Orthostatic (postural) hypotension is common in populations of older people, and rarely has a single cause.

Hypotension may be a feature of shock, where there is inadequate organ perfusion. In this setting, low blood pressure may be accompanied by pallor, air hunger, tachycardia, reduced capillary return and oliguria. Shock may be due to either pump failure or peripheral circulatory failure.

Pump failure includes cardiogenic shock, e.g. secondary to myocardial infarction or secondary as a consequence of pulmonary embolus, tension pneumothorax or cardiac tamponade.

Peripheral circulatory failure can occur due to:

(1)   Hypovolaemia: blood loss, e.g. bleeding peptic ulcer; fluid loss, e.g. severe diarrhoea and vomiting and heat exhaustion;

(2)   Sepsis: severe systemic infection can lead to shock;

(3)   Anaphylaxis, e.g. drug reaction or allergy to peanuts or bee-stings;

(4)   Endocrine disease, e.g. Addison's disease or hypopituitarism;

(5)   Drug side-effects, e.g. antihypertensive overdose.

Shock is a medical emergency. If BP is unrecordable, the cardiac-arrest team should be called. If the patient is hypotensive, immediate help from the medical on-call team should be sought.

The initial management includes:

A   Ascertain 'airway' patency and establish a safe airway;

B   Assess that respiratory rate ('breathing') is adequate – if not, treat as an arrest; check equal and adequate chest wall movement and for signs of pneumothorax; give high-flow oxygen;

C   Check pulse and blood pressure ('circulation') and look for evidence of bleeding.

Elevate the foot of the bed. Gain iv access with two large-bore cannulae and infuse colloid or crystalloid fast to raise blood pressue (providing there is no cardiogenic shock).

Initial investigations should include FBC, urea and electrolytes, glucose, CXR, ECG, arterial blood gases and blood cultures.

Management of patients on psychiatric wards will depend on available local resources and facilities, and speed of access to acute medical care.

Postural hypotension

Postural hypotension is frequently asymptomatic. Dizziness on standing, syncope or fainting and falls may be reported.

Causes of postural hypotension include:

(1)   Hypovolaemia;

(2)   Reduced fluid intake;

(3)   Overtreatment with diuretics;

(4)   Acute haemorrhage;

(5)   Vomiting;

(6)   Diarrhoea;

(7)   Adrenal insufficiency;

(8)   Drugs;

(9)   Diuretics;

(10) Antihypertensives;

(11) Vasodilators;

(12) Antiarrhythmics;

(13) Digoxin;

(14) Psychotropic drugs;

(15) Alcohol;

(16) Anti-parkinsonian drugs.

Autonomic disorders that affect blood flow regulation include:

(1)   Postprandial hypotension;

(2)   Parkinson's disease;

(3)   Multiple system atrophy;

(4)   Uraemia;

(5)   Diabetes mellitus;

(6)   Alcoholism;

(7)   Vitamin B_{12} deficiency.

The clinical situation will often indicate the cause, or at least the major cause, of a problem developing acutely. This underlying cause needs to be treated. In addition, if possible, contributing medications ought to be withdrawn. This can be difficult in practice as the symptoms and the consequences of postural hypotension symptoms must be weighed against the effect of withdrawal of treatment on the underlying condition. Where several drugs are implicated, withdrawal or substitution of a drug with the least impact on the underlying disease should be chosen first and the response to withdrawal on postural hypotension should be monitored. Salt and fluid intake needs to be increased in patients who are not in heart failure. Situations that may exacerbate falls in blood pressure should be avoided (standing for long periods, prolonged recumbency, large meals, hot weather, hot showers and baths). The head of the bed can be elevated to stimulate the renin–angiotensin–aldosterone system, although this is rarely very effective. Pressure hosiery can be effective, but tends not to be well tolerated by patients.

Many drugs have been suggested for the treatment of postural hypotension. Most of these are only moderately effective:

(1)   Caffeine;

(2)   Ephedrine;

(3)   NSAIDs;

(4)   Fludrocortisone;

(5)   Midodrine.

These drugs should not be started by a psychiatrist. Medical help should be sought for advice on treatment. Alcohol and other hypotensive medications should be avoided.

INCONTINENCE: FAECES

Faecal incontinence is the passage of faeces either without awareness or without an ability to control defecation until a socially acceptable time. While rarely curable, it is often manageable, thus averting institutionalisation. The maintenance of continence is complex and involves:

(1) Internal anal sphincter (smooth muscle; prevents faecal leakage);

(2) External anal sphincter (striated muscle; voluntary control);

(3) Anorectal angle (60–105°; > 110° associated with loss of continence);

(4) Anal sensation;

(5) Slit shape of anal canal;

(6) Anal cushions (vascular tissue that closes the anal canal).

When faeces enters the rectum, the anorectal angle increases and the anal sphincters relax (rectoanal inhibitory reflex). Without contraction of the external sphincter, faeces is then expelled by an increase in intra-abdominal pressure.

Incontinence commonly follows damage to the anal sphincters during childbirth or anorectal surgery. Thus, it is predominantly a condition of women. Sometimes it is associated with rectal prolapse. Loose stool may overwhelm the continence mechanisms and cause incontinence. In those with dementia, there may be loss of awareness of 'the call to stool' and a failure to inhibit defaecation; uninhibited contractions may be sufficient to expel soft, but not hard, stool.

The history should record, if possible, the number and types of vaginal deliveries and any past history of anorectal surgery. Also, the pattern of faecal incontinence needs to be determined: bowel charts will aid this. In women, urinary incontinence is often also present as part of pelvic floor weakness. Always check the drug chart for excessive laxative administration. Evidence of damage to sacral nerve roots needs to be sought. The patient also requires a rectal examination and assessment of anal sphincter tone and force of contraction (page 56).

Management of faecal incontinence in the setting of significant dementia usually differs from that in the cognitively intact individual. For the patient with significant dementia, the issue is one of containment. In essence, one is trying to induce defaecation at a time that is convenient, and, if necessary, to suppress it at other times. This can usually be achieved with a combination of stimulant laxatives interspersed with constipating drugs. In addition, enemas may also be needed.

In the non-demented patient, it is advisable to seek advice as newer surgical procedures may be feasible. If a rectal prolapse is present, it is advised to refer for surgical management.

INCONTINENCE: URINE

Urinary incontinence is reported to occur in 16% of elderly women and 8% of elderly men. Incontinence is a symptom which must be evaluated.

In infants, the bladder fills and empties in a reflex manner. Continence occurs with the development of afferent pathways to sense bladder fullness, and inhibitory efferent pathways to suppress reflex bladder emptying.

Incontinence occurs when the bladder pressure is increased through increased bladder contraction, through urinary retention or when urethral closing pressure is reduced.

Patterns of urinary incontinence

Urge incontinence is seen with bladder/detrusor instability. Typically there is loss of large volumes of urine accompanied by a sensation of urgency. It can be associated with neurological disease, e.g. stroke, multiple sclerosis.

Stress incontinence is usually seen in women, and occasionally in men post-prostatectomy. Typically there is loss of small volumes of urine which occur with manoeuvres that raise intra-abdominal pressure, e.g. coughing or straining.

Overflow incontinence is where there is constant involuntary leakage of small volumes of urine. This occurs where there is reduced bladder contraction or outflow obstruction. It is commonly seen in men with prostatic hypertrophy, but is also seen in patients with constipation or as a side-effect of drugs with anticholinergic activity. Symptoms of poor stream or flow, the need to strain to pass urine or a sensation of incomplete emptying may be reported. More rarely, bladder fistulae may lead to constant urine leakage.

Functional incontinence is a term used for those who would usually be continent but, because of physical problems, cognitive problems or the use of medication, are unable to reach toilet facilities in time. Examples include decreased mobility due to severe arthritis, and high-dose diuretic therapy in a poorly mobile patient. This is a common problem for elderly patients admitted to hospital.

Investigation

If symptoms are mild and not bothersome to the patient, then no action may be required. Referral via the General Practitioner (GP) for a community continence assessment can be suggested. Continence that has previously been evaluated may need no further action.

Many psychiatrists may not feel either confident or competent, particularly with pelvic examination, and may wish to refer for the assessment of continence. Many hospitals now have trained nurses as continence advisors who will help. Referral to a gynaecologist, urologist or a geriatrician may be considered.

Reversible causes of urinary incontinence should be considered and treated. These can be described by the mnemonic DRIPP: delirium; restricted mobility; infection (acute symptomatic urinary tract infection), impaction of stool, inflammation (atrophic vaginitis); polyuria (diabetes mellitus, caffeine intake, volume overload); pharmacological (diuretics, psychotropics, anticholinergics).

The continence history should determine the onset and duration of continence, day and night frequency and pattern, awareness of continence and the presence of any precipitants. Volume intake and voiding symptoms such as dysuria straining, haematuria, urgency, hesitancy and poor stream should be elicited. Voiding charts recording timing and volumes of incontinence are helpful in determining patterns of incontinence. Review medications to see whether any are aggravating incontinence. Relevant previous illnesses such as neurological disease, diabetes mellitus, abdominal surgery, prostate surgery or pelvic irradiation should be determined.

Examination should include an assessment of cognitive function, abdominal examination for palpable bladder or faecal masses. Rectal examination should assess prostate size in men, the presence of faecal impaction and anal tone and perianal sensation. Inspection of the external genitalia may reveal phimosis in men, or evidence of ammoniacal dermatitis suggesting prolonged incontinence. In women, vaginal examination is required to detect prolapse, cystocoele and atrophic vaginitis. A neurological examination is required to determine evidence of stroke, peripheral neuropathy or cord compression.

There is a poor relationship between positive urine cultures and long-standing urinary incontinence. However, new-onset incontinence may be related to infection, and urine should be dipstick tested and sent for culture if positive. Consider one course of treatment for urinary infection. Urea and electrolytes, glucose and calcium should be checked. Check prostate-specific antigen (PSA) in men with prostatic symptoms.

Residual volume should be measured, ideally using a bladder scan; a continence nurse may provide this service. Alternatively, a clean, diagnostic, post-void catheterisation for measurement of residual volume can be made. Whilst there are no fixed guidelines on residual volume, a volume > 150 ml may need further investigation.

Management

With treatment, 70% of patients may be cured or their symptoms improved. The following general measures can improve continence:

(1)   Limit fluid intake to 1.5 l/day;

(2)   Reduce caffeine and alcohol intake;

(3)   Treat aggravating factors such as infection, constipation or cough;

(4)   Review medication and reduce or eliminate offending drugs.

Specific treatments

Urge incontinence

(1)   Individual toileting programme and bladder training;

(2)   Anticholinergic medication, e.g. oxybutynin or tolterodine (NB this should not be used in individuals with raised residual volumes).

Stress incontinence

(1)   Pelvic floor exercises;

(2)   Electrical stimulation;

(3)   Local oestrogens;

(4)   Surgical interventions (refer to gynaecology/urology).

Overflow incontinence

(1)   Alpha-blockers;

(2)   Surgery for benign prostatic hypertrophy (refer to urologist).

Containment methods

A continence advisor will provide guidance on the use of:

(1) Pads;

(2) Urinals;

(3) Bedding.

INFECTION: GENERAL

Infections are very common at all ages, including old age. Whether or not there are age-related changes in host defence mechanisms, including the immune response, is still uncertain. In fact, the inflammatory responses of old people are more likely to be exaggerated than depressed, and this may contribute to tissue injury and morbidity (adult respiratory distress syndrome, systemic inflammatory response syndrome): aging can be viewed as a hyperinflammatory state. Epidemiological studies related to this topic are often unsatisfactory, and the best ones show the least effects of old age. It is best to consider that old age is not a generally immune-compromised state predisposing to infections, but rather, a state in which infections are commoner at certain sites (e.g. urinary infections).

To acquire an infection, there must be exposure to the pathogen. The potential pathogen must then proliferate, usually at some mucosal surface. The outcome of this may be elimination of the pathogen, colonisation by the pathogen (when host defences fail to eliminate the pathogen but are sufficient to prevent tissue invasion) or tissue invasion. For most infections, tissue invasion is required for a state of infection to exist: some organisms cause illness by releasing toxins without tissue invasion (usually diarrhoeal illnesses). There are genetic factors too which determine the outcome of the encounter between host and pathogen. A good example is that not all people have the receptors on their enteric mucosal cells to allow some viral agents that cause diarrhoea to enter the cells: not all patients exposed to such pathogens will acquire the illness, regardless of infection control measures.

Systemic illness, undernutrition and general debilitation certainly predispose to infections, especially those caused by bacterial pathogens. Still, in order to acquire such a pathogen, exposure to it must occur. Exposure is much more likely in closed communities where people have frequent contact with others (hospitals, nursing homes). In particular, medical, nursing and other ward staff can act as vectors for these pathogens. The single most effective measure to prevent such transmission is for you (and them) to wash your hands both before and after having physical contact with any patient.

The recognition that an infection is present (other than those organisms that elaborate toxins) will be determined by recognising the host response (cough, sputum production, diarrhoea, dysuria, fever, raised white cell count, raised levels of inflammatory markers, etc.). For most (but not all) old people, these host responses function perfectly well, although they may be masked by co-morbid factors. Thus, you need to search for them carefully.

The outcome of infections usually differs significantly between young and old people. However, in the 1918 influenza pandemic, it was younger people who died rather than older ones. The reasons for the exaggerated mortality of aging relate partly to the exaggerated inflammatory response (causing exaggerated tissue injury and organ failure) and a failure of reserve capacities in many organ systems that lead to premature decompensation, more severe illness and possibly death. In those who survive, recovery after a serious infection can be very prolonged.

INFECTION: URINARY TRACT

Urinary tract infection is common in the elderly, and the incidence rises with advancing age. Clinical features of lower urinary tract infection include frequency, dysuria and urgency. Infection of the upper renal tract may include symptoms of loin pain, fever and rigors. In the elderly it may not be possible to distinguish upper from lower urinary infection.

Urinary infection is usually diagnosed by the presence of 'significant bacteriuria': $> 10^5$ organisms/ml in a mid-stream specimen of urine. However 'significant bacteriuria' is frequently asymptomatic in the elderly. If used as the sole criterion of infection, 20% of community-dwelling elderly women and 10% of elderly men have an infection. Almost one-third of acute elderly medical admissions have 'significant bacteriuria'. In nursing-home residents the prevalence of significant bacteriuria is recorded as 30–50%. Collection of urine samples is technically difficult in frail and confused patients, and samples are frequently contaminated.

The atypical or 'geriatric presentation' with fatigue, malaise, confusion or falls is frequently ascribed to urinary infection. Given the high prevalence of asymptomatic bacteriuria, how can causation be established? Asymptomatic bacteriuria remits and recurs spontaneously, is associated with a low incidence of the development of symptomatic disease and is poorly correlated with symptoms of general well-being. Bacteriuria has not been found to predict mortality in elderly women, and antibiotic treatment does not reduce mortality.

How should clinical practice reflect these findings? First, routine urine culture should be abandoned. Urine culture should be limited to symptomatic subjects, i.e. those with dysuria. Dipstick testing of urine may precede culture. A negative dipstick test for white cells, or the absence of pyuria on microscopy, are highly predictive of a negative culture. The urinary tract is a frequent source of bacteraemia and a low index of suspicion is needed. Blood cultures should be performed if there is evidence of systemic illness and in patients suspected to have pyelonephritis. Whilst in younger patients, pyelonephritis may prompt investigation for structural abnormalities of the urinary tract, this is not the case in most elderly female patients, and in elderly men, investigation for structural abnormalities should be tempered by the likelihood of the patient attaining benefit from investigation and treatment.

Many older patients have indwelling urinary catheters. Urine is colonised within days of catheterisation and patients are asymptomatic. Catheter-related sepsis is a frequent cause of bacteraemia, especially if catheter blockage occurs. As urine colonisation is ubiquitous in catheterised patients, urine infection is not always the cause of fever and illness and other potential sources should be sought. Treatment should be guided by blood cultures in addition to urine culture.

Treatment

Lower urinary tract infection should be treated with oral antibiotics. Most hospitals produce formularies to guide treatment, which is usually given for 3–5 days in women and for 7–10 days in men. Patients suspected of having upper urinary tract infection usually require intravenous antibiotics initially, and should be transferred to a geriatric or medical ward. Treatment is usually given for 10–14 days.

ITCH

Background

Itch or pruritus is a skin sensation leading to the desire to scratch. Tissue damage caused by scratching may lead to acute conditions such as scratch prurigo (itchy wheals from scratching) or to chronic lichenified patches known as prurigo nodularis. Most acute and chronic skin diseases produce some itch.

Itch in normal-appearing skin may be a feature of systemic disease. In the elderly especially, itch may occur in normal-appearing skin in the absence of systemic disease. In this setting the itching is thought to be due to reduced water content of the skin without evident dryness. Itching without skin changes is also seen in that caused by water – aquagenic pruritus. Common skin rashes affecting older people are described on page 181.

The pathophysiology of itch is poorly understood. Like pain, itch may be peripheral in origin (dermal or neuropathic) or central (neuropathic, neurogenic, psychogenic).

Clinical assessment

No rash except scaling or dry skin

The most likely diagnosis in the elderly is dry skin (xerosis), sometimes called 'senile pruritus'. Try moisturising (emollient) creams such as aqueous cream. Sometimes menthol or phenol are added to emollients. Frequent bathing can aggravate symptoms. Sedative antihistamines may be given if sleep is disturbed or symptoms are troublesome.

Other causes to consider include:

(1) Systemic disease:

    (a) Liver disease (check liver function tests);

    (b) Uraemia (check urea and electrolytes, creatinine);

    (c) Polycythaemia (haemoglobin);

    (d) Anaemia (iron deficiency, check ferritin);

(2) Malignancy: general examination for lymph nodes, masses, liver and spleen, CXR;

(3) Endocrine causes: hypo- and hyperthyroidism, hyperparathyroidism (check thyroid function tests, calcium);

(4) Drugs: itch can occur without rash as a drug side-effect, e.g. opiates and drugs causing cholestasis, e.g. phenothiazines;

(5) Infestation: scabies (usually seen with rash), body lice;

(6) Irritants: wool clothing, especially in atopic patients;

(7)   Psychogenic itch: symptoms typically when patients are not occupied, does not wake from sleep.

Rash is present with itching

All rashes may itch to some degree. Common causes of itching rash are eczema/dermatitis and urticaria (visible wheals). Fungal rashes in the groin (intertrigo) may be itchy. Scabies is one of the commonest causes of itch, especially in institutionalised patients. Drug reactions (page 184) may produce an itchy rash whose onset can often be related to a new drug prescription.

Scabies

The typical lesion is a burrow, a linear ridge often ending in a tiny vesicle. Usually they are seen in the interdigital web spaces, axillae, umbilicus, genitalia and volar aspects of the wrists. Papules, vesicles, nodules and excoriations may also be seen. Although the diagnosis can be confirmed by scrapings of a burrow content onto a slide for microscopy, the diagnosis is usually made clinically. Treatment is with permethrim cream or malathion liquid in an aqueous base. Treatment is often recommended for close contacts and household members. The itching is due to a hypersensitivity reaction and can persist after treatment is completed.

Getting help

Diagnosing rashes can be difficult in elderly patients – for geriatricians too! Advice from a dermatologist may be required.

NAUSEA AND VOMITING

Vomiting is the means by which the upper gut rids itself of its contents when almost any part is irritated, distended or 'irritable'. The irritation or distension of the duodenum seems to be a particularly potent stimulus. Signals are conveyed by both vagal and sympathetic afferents to bilaterally represented vomiting centres in the medulla. Nausea is a conscious recognition of the subconscious activation of this area. Vomiting is usually, but not always, preceded by nausea. The motor output that causes vomiting is carried in cranial nerves V, VII, IX, X and XII to the upper gut, abdominal muscles and diaphragm.

The first event is usually antiperistalsis, which may begin far along the ileum. This distends the duodenum over several minutes before the act of vomiting occurs. The lower oesophageal sphincter relaxes, and contractions of the stomach and duodenum convey the contents to the oesophagus. Then, the act of vomiting is triggered. There is a deep breath, the hyoid bone and the larynx are elevated and the glottis closes. Then, strong contractions of the abdominal muscles expel the upper gut contents to the outside.

Not all vomiting is induced by local causes in the upper gut. It can also be induced by stimulation of the chemoreceptor trigger zone in the floor of the fourth ventricle. Stimulation can be direct (drugs, chemicals) or indirect (vestibular labyrinth, higher centres). Higher centres are usually the trigger for vomiting in response to bad smells, disgusting sights, etc.

Causes of nausea and vomiting

The above review of the physiology of vomiting and nausea shows the causes to be local upper-gastrointestinal (GI) disorders, stimulation of the chemoreceptor trigger zone or vomiting centres directly (usually drugs and toxins) and stimulation from higher centres (e.g. unpleasant sights, bad smells, etc.). In your practice, the commonest cause will be medications. Other causes include:

(1) Gastroenteritis;

(2) Non-GI infections (e.g. urinary infection, pneumonia);

(3) Persistent coughing;

(4) Acute labyrinthitis;

(5) Peptic ulcer disease;

(6) Gastritis;

(7) Gall-bladder disease;

(8) Electrolyte disorders;

(9) Hyperglycaemia (and hypoglycaemia);

(10) Uraemia;

(11) Intestinal obstruction;

(12) Migraine;

(13) Acute angle closure glaucoma;

(14) Severe constipation;

(15) Raised intracranial pressure.

The patient merits a careful assessment aimed at noting any associated symptoms that point to any of the conditions listed above. Physical examination should focus on these, particularly the abdomen. The drug chart needs to be reviewed, and the drugs should be looked up in the BNF to see whether nausea and vomiting are known side-effects.

Antiemetics

Nausea should never be treated symptomatically without a determined attempt to find the cause. The underlying cause, where possible, must be treated. Drugs used for the symptomatic management of nausea include:

(1)   Antihistamines (variably effective);

(2)   Phenothiazines (act on chemoreceptor trigger zone);

(3)   Metoclopramide;

(4)   Domperidone;

(5)   Ondansetron (acts peripherally and centrally).

NOSEBLEEDS

Nosebleeds are commonest in the very young and the very old. You may encounter it as a recurrent problem or as a new problem, with the patient unable to control the bleeding. This situation is alarming, but it is only very rarely life-threatening. The causes include:

(1)   Spontaneous from Little's area (exacerbated by nose-picking);

(2)   Trauma;

(3)   Nasal infection;

(4)   Drugs (especially anticoagulants);

(5)   Hypertension;

(6)   Septal inflammation;

(7) Thrombocytopenia;

(8) Tumours;

(9) Leukaemia;

(10) Vitamin K deficiency;

(11) Liver failure.

History

This is indicated from the above list of causes. Particularly, check whether the patient is taking anticoagulants.

Examination

Check the blood pressure. A detailed examination is usually not required unless suggested by the history. If there is widespread bruising associated with the nosebleed, check the prothrombin time and platelet count.

Management

Apply local pressure with gauze pads or cotton wool: the bleeding should stop. If it does not, or it recurs, get an ENT opinion. If this is not immediately available, discuss the patient with the local A&E department.

PAIN

Psychiatrists will encounter pain in two main circumstances:

(1) A patient under your care complains of pain;

(2) A patient is referred for an opinion about whether the pain has a psychogenic origin.

From a traditional medical perspective, pain is a signal of some underlying disease or disorder: the focus is on the nature of the underlying disorder rather than on the patient suffering the pain. Thus, there will be an investigation(s) to determine the nature of the underlying cause(s). This is, depending on circumstances, a valid approach, but only up to a point. When efforts to elicit the underlying cause(s) fail, or the treatment proves inadequate, patients may then be labelled as untreatable and the patient is still left with the symptom. Physicians tend to attribute the pain to an organic cause when a suitable underlying physical explanation is found, and to label it as psychogenic when a physical cause cannot be adequately defined, or, if it can, the pain seems disproportionate to the underlying disorder or the treatment is not as effective as they think it ought to be.

The recognition that pain treatment, especially of chronic pain, is often inadequate and disappointing has led to a broader conceptualisation of the nature of pain, and a biopsychosocial model is generally applied in specialist pain treatment services. Its focus is on the notion that the biological nature of pain is just a part of what a patient experiences, and more effective interventions are possible when psychological and social factors are recognised and utilised in the management of pain. Thus, medications and physical methods provide only part of a solution for many patients.

The neuroanatomy of pain

Pain, in a biological context, is the unpleasant sensory experience associated with actual or potential tissue damage, or is described in terms of such damage. Pain occurs when nociceptors are stimulated, but may also be felt in the absence of such stimulation. Up to 50% of community-dwelling elderly subjects report pain. Aging does not change pain perception apart from some reduction in visceral pain sensation. For example, pain may not be reported with an acute myocardial infarction, or experienced with an acute abdominal disorder. Pain perception may be raised with co-existing depression (complicates many somatic illnesses), which should be sought and treated.

Neuroanatomically, painful stimuli activate A-delta (myelinated) and C (unmyelinated) fibres, whose long dendrites extend to skin, muscle, connective tissues, joints, bone and internal organs. Other, non-pain-mediating A-beta (myelinated) fibres carry localisation information, although the viscera lack this type of innervation and localisation is generally poor. All three types of neurons relay in the dorsal horn of the spinal cord, either directly or indirectly (through interneurons), with second-order neurons. Facial pain relays through the trigeminal nerve to second-order neurons in the pons and medulla.

In the spinal cord, the second-order neurons originate in laminae I, II and V of the dorsal horn, where the A-delta and C fibres terminate. The substantia gelatinosa of lamina II undertakes considerable modulation via interneurons that serve as gates or switches through which the information being conducted is either enhanced or suppressed. This may explain why local strategies such as rubbing or cutaneous nerve stimulation suppress pain – a phenomenon often called counter-irritation. The substantia gelatinosa receives extensive serotonergic and adrenergic innervation from the brain, further modulating the sensation of pain.

Not all of the cells in these laminae of the dorsal horn are pain-specific. Some neurons fire at different frequencies according to whether or not the stimulus is nociceptive (wide dynamic range or WDR cells). The lamina V WDR cells receive both visceral and non-visceral input, which explains the phenomenon of referred pain. For example, nociception in the heart is often perceived in the left neck, left shoulder and left arm as well as in the chest.

Most of the axons arising from the second-order neurons cross the anterior commissure to ascend in the anterolateral spinal white matter to terminate in the thalamus, although a small number of fibres ascend ipsilaterally. These axons terminate either in the ventroposterior thalamic nucleus (neospinothalamic system) or in the medial thalamic nucleus (paleospinothalamic system). Third-order neurons of the neospinothalamic system relay to the sensory cortex of the parietal lobe (localisation and coordination of the motor response). Those of the paleospinothalamic system relay to the reticular formation, hypothalamus and prefrontal cortex. These two pathways give rise to the autonomic, affective and cognitive responses to the painful stimulus.

CNS modulation of pain

Four brain regions are involved in reducing pain:

(1)   Cortex and limbic structures;

(2)   Mid-brain (PAG: peri-aqueductal grey matter);

(3)   Rostroventral medulla (RVM; projects to laminae I, II and V of spinal dorsal horn);

(4)   Spinal dorsal horn.

Opiates activate μ opioid receptors in the peri-aqueductal grey matter and RVM. The PAG relays to neighbouring serotonergic (RVM) and adrenergic (dorsolateral pons) structures.

There are also CNS mechanisms that can augment pain, and these may promote chronicity. It is well established that inadequate treatment of acute pain promotes the emergence of chronic pain. These include ongoing peripheral (often inflammatory) stimuli, alterations in peripheral nerves, altered motor activity, dorsal horn sensitisation (associated with glutamate and NMDA (*N*-methyl-D-asparate) receptor activation), sympathetic nervous system activation and changes in the limbic system and cerebral cortex.

Chemicals and neurotransmitters involved in pain

Pain-augmenting chemicals active at a site of injury include:

(1) Kinins;

(2) Histamine;

(3) Serotonin;

(4) Potassium;

(5) Prostaglandins.

Neurotransmitters increasing pain include:

(1) Substance P;

(2) Glutamate.

Pain-inhibiting neurotransmitters include:

(1) Opioids (mainly via μ receptors);

(2) Adrenergic agonists;

(3) Serotonin;

(4) Neurotensin.

Acute versus chronic pain

Acute pain is a beneficial response to preserve life and limb. Usually, acute pain disappears with resolution of the initial stimulus. However, sometimes it does not, and it may even seem to take on a life of its own. Sometimes, this aberrant response occurs frequently and predictably, as in phantom limb pain and in post-herpetic neuralgia following an attack of shingles. One risk factor known to predispose to the development of chronicity is a failure adequately to control pain acutely. In the literature on pain, acute pain is that which is present within 6 months of the precipitating stimulus, and chronic pain is that which is present after 6 months. However, this definition is not entirely satisfactory, and other associated factors need to be considered before deciding on a treatment approach.

Chronic pain has been classified as nociceptive (both somatic and visceral), neuropathic (includes central nervous system) or psychogenic (no clear underlying cause). Chronic pain tends to have pervasive effects on function and affect (the extent varying with differing personalities). It is further complicated by secondary effects on relationships and life-style, as well as by ongoing litigation. It is beyond our remit to go into detail about these consequences of pain, and you will need to look elsewhere for more information.

The treatment of pain

Often, acute pain is not well managed, even in situations where you might expect that it should be well managed, as the pain is predictable (e.g. after hip fracture surgery). The reasons for this are not well understood, but are likely to include a failure to appreciate that there is a problem, a failure to assess pain severity adequately and a failure to prescribe the right drugs in the right doses.

A hierarchy of analgesics is often recommended in treating painful conditions, and the choice of drug depends on the severity of the pain, and the treatment is changed according to the response. We recommend that you always choose the least invasive route of administration that is feasible. Note that there is often a large placebo response in trials of analgesics. For mild–moderate acute pain, paracetamol is often used as a starting drug, except for those with liver disease. It must also be used with caution in those on warfarin. The most useful measure of the efficacy of analgesics that is widely reported in trials and systematic reviews is the number needed to treat (NNT), compared with a placebo and/or another drug, to produce at least a 50% reduction in the perceived pain. In the acute setting, using single doses, trials reveal an NNT for paracetamol of about 4.5: this means that one in five patients will get at least 50% pain reduction who would not have done so if they had received only the placebo. Adding codeine (60 mg) to paracetamol produces an extra response over paracetamol alone for every eight patients treated. In similar studies, the NSAID diclofenac produces an NNT of 2.6, a figure that is very similar to that produced by 10 mg of morphine. Thus, in our hierarchy, diclofenac (50 mg) = morphine (10 mg) > paracetamol (1000 mg) > codeine (60 mg).

All other things being equal, we recommend paracetamol for mild–moderate acute pain and, if the response is not adequate, to add diclofenac or nefopam. If the response is still inadequate, substitute a strong opioid. Indeed, we feel that strong opioids are underused in the setting of acute pain management, which is a pity because they are generally safe and effective. We do not recommend using codeine because of the universality and severity of the associated constipation. Do not combine weak and strong opioids, as the weak ones may reduce the effect of the strong one.

For chronic pain, the World Health Organization recommends the use of a pain management ladder, originally recommended for cancer pain. Start with a non-opioid and add a weak opioid if the response is inadequate. If this does not produce an adequate response, substitute a strong opioid for the weak one. If this is ineffective or side-effects limit dose increases, other approaches are indicated. It may be best to seek advice at this stage. Other approaches include:

(1)   Antidepressants;

(2)   Anticonvulsants;

(3)   Local anaesthesia (local anaesthetic, opioid);

(4)   Nerve destruction;

(5)   Surgery;

(6)   Radiotherapy (bone metastases);

(7)   Transcutaneous electrical nerve stimulation (TENS);

(8)   Acupuncture;

(9)   Psychological interventions;

(10) Hypnosis.

Antidepressants and anticonvulsants are most often used to treat neuropathic pain. Tricyclic antidepressants seem to be more effective than SSRIs in this regard. There is no truth in the old adage 'treat burning pain with an antidepressant and shooting pain with an anticonvulsant'. It is not clear whether combining an antidepressant with an anticonvulsant produces greater pain relief. We do not yet know which is the best antidepressant or anticonvulsant to treat neuropathic pain.

Paracetamol

Paracetamol, a derivative of aniline, is probably the most widely prescribed analgesic for mild–moderate acute and chronic pain, for which it is effective. It is also antipyretic. Its site of action remains unknown, but is most likely in the CNS. It is rapidly absorbed when given orally, and has a plasma half-life of about 2 hours. The dose schedule is 0.5–1 g every 4–6 hours up to a maximum of 4 g per day for short-term treatment. When used for longer-term treatment, it is recommended that the maximum daily dose should be 3 g. It is available as tablets, capsules, suppositories and liquid formulations. It is relatively free of side-effects and drug interactions, although it is very toxic to the liver in overdose; paracetamol overdose is a medical emergency. Its hepatotoxicity is exacerbated by alcohol. It also reduces the dose of warfarin needed to achieve anticoagulation targets.

Non-steroidal anti-inflammatory drugs

These drugs are anti-inflammatory, analgesic and antipyretic. Like aspirin, they inhibit cyclo-oxygenase (COX), which is a key enzyme in E-series prostaglandin production. They also inhibit some other enzymes such as phospholipase-C in macrophages. Their main indication is for pain with an inflammatory component. COX-1 is constitutively expressed in many tissues whereas COX-2 is not (except in parts of the brain and a few other sites). COX-2 is induced at sites of inflammation and in some cancers. All non-selective NSAIDs inhibit both enzymes, which explains their toxicity (gastrointestinal bleeding, nephrotoxicity, fluid retention). All are lipophilic and cross the blood–brain barrier: they can sometimes cause stupor, delirium and mood changes, occasionally after a single dose). They also tend to elevate blood lithium levels (sulindac is less problematic in this regard). Thus, they should be avoided or used with care in patients with peptic ulceration, renal disease, heart disease, liver disease and those taking lithium. Older people have an enhanced susceptibility to such toxicity, so you should always think twice before using them at all, and you should co-prescribe gastric-protecting drugs such as proton pump inhibitors (well tolerated) or misoprostol (not well tolerated). If you decide to use NSAIDs, watch carefully for signs of toxicity and try to avoid long-term use, if at all possible.

The problem of toxicity led to the search for selective inhibitors of COX-2, which cannot now be recommended owing to the development of an increased risk of stroke.

Most NSAIDs are completely absorbed with oral administration, although the absorption rate may vary. Plasma half-life varies according to preparation, and those with a long half-life (and usually slower absorption) are not recommended for acute pain management (e.g. piroxicam). Diclofenac has the shortest half-life, and it is the one we recommend in geriatric practice for patients not taking lithium. Diclofenac is available as 25-mg tablets, and the daily dose is 75–150 mg given in 2–3 divided doses.

There is a combination tablet which includes misoprostol (200 mg) and diclofenac (50 mg), one tablet 2–3 times daily. Diclofenac is also available in sustained-release form, and there is an injectable formulation. If the patient is taking lithium, sulindac is perhaps a safer choice. It is a pro-drug available as 100-mg tablets to be given twice daily. The maximum daily dose is 400 mg.

Nefopam

Nefopam is a non-opioid analgesic whose mechanism of action is not fully understood, but it is likely to be in the CNS. It has a rapid onset of action, and it is more effective than paracetamol or NSAIDs in relieving pain. It is useful for both acute and chronic pain. Sympathomimetic and anticholinergic side-effects limit its use. Side-effects, which are dose-related, include:

(1)   Difficulty in passing urine (urinary retention);

(2)   Dry mouth;

(3)   Nausea and vomiting;

(4)   Light-headedness;

(5)   Nervousness;

(6)   Delirium;

(7)   Psychosis;

(8)   Increased heart rate (tachycardia);

(9)   Headache;

(10) Blurred vision;

(11) Difficulty in sleeping (insomnia);

(12) Drowsiness;

(13) Sweating;

(14) Seizures;

(15) Pink urine.

It should not be used in patients with epilepsy, those on tricyclic antidepressants or those taking MAOIs. Alcohol should be avoided as it increases sedation. In our experience, most older patients tolerate 30 mg 8-hourly, and very few tolerate the maximum dose of 90 mg 8-hourly. Patients vary in their ability to tolerate 60 mg 8-hourly.

Opioid analgesics

The term opioid refers to all agonists with morphine-like pharmacological activity that can be antagonised by the opioid antagonist, naloxone. Both complete and partial agonists are known. Complete agonists are also called strong opioids or high-efficacy opioids, as they need only occupy a minority of available receptors (10–20%) to produce a maximum pharmacological response. Partial opioid agonists (weak opioids, low-efficacy opioids) need to occupy most of the available receptors (75–100%) to produce a maximum response. Weak agonists can displace strong agonists from opioid receptors, thereby reducing analgesia.

Three families of opioid receptors are currently recognised: μ, δ and κ. The μ_1 receptors mediate supraspinal analgesia, sedation, euphoria, nausea and emesis. The μ_2 receptors mediate spinal analgesia, respiratory depression and constipation. Most commercially available opioids are either complete or partial μ receptor agonists, although some activate other receptors too. Codeine (weak) and morphine (strong) have δ agonist activity. Pentazocine has some κ agonist activity. Tramadol, as well as being a μ receptor agonist, also antagonises the reuptake of noradrenaline and serotonin: it should not be used for patients taking MAOIs. Naloxone blocks all three classes of receptors and has no agonist activity: it is used to treat opioid overdose.

There are many opioids available, and we suggest that you become familiar with a small number. Your local hospital guidelines may differ from our preferences, so it is difficult for us to make recommendations. Laxatives will usually be needed by patients taking opioids; antiemetics will often be needed when using strong opioids. We list below some commonly available weak and strong opioids, and indicate with an asterisk the ones we tend to use.

Weak opioids

(1)   Codeine;

(2)   Dihydrocodeine (sustained-release preparation: DHC Continus®);

(3)   Oxycodone (sustained-release preparation: OxyContin®)*;

(4)   Pentazocine;

(5)   Tramadol (sustained-release preparation: several choices)*.

Strong opioids

(1)   Morphine (sustained-release preparation available)*;

(2)   Diamorphine (highly potent: small injection volume);

(3)   Dextromoramide (short-acting; useful for breakthrough pain);

(4)   Hydromorphone (sustained-release preparation: Palladone® SR)*;

(5)   Methadone;

(6)   Fentanyl (transdermal, long-acting preparation: Durogesic®)*;

(7)   Phenazocine (highly potent: small injection volume).

Antidepressants

These are useful for three reasons:

(1)   Direct analgesic effects (independent of effects on mood);

(2)   To treat associated depression;

(3)   To improve sleep and appetite disturbances caused by pain.

The analgesia induced by antidepressants is thought to be mediated by enhancing the inhibitory neurotransmitters (noradrenaline and serotonin) of the descending pain pathways. They may also augment opioid analgesia at the spinal level. Tricyclic antidepressants are generally avoided for older patients owing to their increased susceptibility to side-effects. SSRIs and venlafaxine are more often used, and the choice of drug often depends on whether sedation will be beneficial or not.

Anticonvulsants

The aberrant sodium channel activity believed to be associated with many neuropathic pains suggests that many anticonvulsants may be useful for treatment. Most anticonvulsants have multiple pharmacological effects that may benefit the treatment of neuropathic pain (GABA enhancement, calcium channel blockade and reduction of excitatory amino acids).

While most experience has been gained using carbamazepine, gabapentin is becoming the anticonvulsant of choice as it is much better tolerated and it elevates mood. The commonest side-effects include sedation, dizziness, fatigue, nystagmus, tremor, nausea and vomiting. The drug is usually given as 300 mg on day one, 300 mg twice daily on day two and 300 mg thrice daily on day three. This rapid dose increase schedule can minimise the duration of troublesome side-effects. The dose is then changed by 300 mg daily (in divided doses) according to response. It is available as capsules of varying strength (100 mg, 300 mg, 400 mg) and as 600-mg tablets. The usual maximum dose is 2400 mg per day. Gabapentin is eliminated in the urine and the dose needs to be reduced according to the glomerular filtration rate: the manufacturer's leaflet tells you how to do this. Do not stop gabapentin abruptly!

Carbamazepine is predominantly a sodium channel blocker. It is metabolised in the liver and it induces its own metabolism (autoinduction). It is available as 100-mg, 200-mg and 400-mg tablets, 100-mg and 200-mg chewtabs, 100-mg/5 ml liquid and 125 mg suppositories. The starting dose is 100 mg twice daily, and most patients can be managed with less than 800 mg per day. Dose adjustments should not be made at less than weekly intervals. The maximum dose you should use is 1600 mg per day. It has extensive interactions with other drugs, especially other anticonvulsants. Side-effects include aplastic anaemia, leukopaenia, rash (occasionally Stevens–Johnson syndrome), hyponatraemia, myoclonus, nausea, vomiting, dizziness and sedation.

We recommend gabapentin as the first-line agent for older people and carbamazepine as the second-line treatment. At present, there is no evidence that other anticonvulsants will be more appropriate.

Other drugs used to treat pain

Although we advise that you do not use them, there are several other medications employed in pain management:

(1)　Antihistamines;

(2)　Benzodiazepines;

(3)　Methylphenidate;

(4)　Neuroleptics;

(5)　Mexiletine;

(6)　α-Adrenoreceptor antagonists;

(7)　Ketamine;

(8)   Glucocorticoids;

(9)   Baclofen;

(10) Capsaicin.

PAIN: ABDOMEN

Acute pain

The sudden onset of severe abdominal pain should always be taken seriously. If the patient is obviously unwell, further deterioration can occur rapidly. The situation is further complicated by the possibility of atypical presentations in older people. For almost all of the likely causes we list below, you will need to refer the patient for further advice and management. Essentially, the decision you need to make is whether to refer to a physician/geriatrician or to a surgeon and how urgent the situation is.

Commoner causes

(1)   Peptic ulcer disease;

(2)   Perforated viscus;

(3)   Oesophagitis;

(4)   Biliary colic;

(5)   Cholecystitis/cholangitis;

(6)   Appendicitis;

(7)   Mesenteric ischaemia;

(8)   Gastroenteritis;

(9)   Renal colic;

(10) Pyelonephritis;

(11) Diverticulitis;

(12) Bowel obstruction;

(13) Pancreatitis;

(14) Ilioinguinal neuralgia;

(15) Genitofemoral neuralgia.

Rarer causes

(1)   Oesophageal dysmotility;

(2)   Shingles (pain precedes rash);

(3)   Hepatitis;

(4)   Inflammatory bowel disease;

(5)   Leaking or dissecting aneurysm;

(6)   Myocardial infarction;

(7)   Acute renal infarction (flank pain);

(8)   Diabetic ketoacidosis;

(9)   Pneumonia.

Pain that is instantaneous in onset suggests a perforated ulcer, aneurysmal dissection/leak or myocardial infarction. Severe, constant pain suggests pancreatitis.

Chronic/recurrent abdominal pain

Chronic and recurrent pain is generally less urgent a problem than acute abdominal pain, and the likely underlying causes are different.

Commoner causes

(1)   Peptic ulcer disease;

(2)   GORD;

(3)   Constipation (page 75);

(4)   Subacute obstruction (adhesions, cancer);

(5)   Diverticular disease;

(6)   Gallstones.

Rarer causes

(1)   Post-herpetic neuralgia;

(2)   Hydronephrosis;

(3)   Inflammatory bowel disease;

(4)   Mesenteric ischaemia;

(5)   Chronic pancreatitis;

(6)   Addison's disease.

Clinical history with abdominal pain

Epigastric pain suggests peptic ulcer disease, oesophagitis, pancreatitis or myocardial infarction. Right upper-quadrant pain points to gall-bladder disease, liver disease, pancreatic disease and pneumonia. Right lower-quadrant pain points to the appendix and caecum and left lower-quadrant pain points to the sigmoid colon and rectum (e.g. diverticulitis). Mid-abdominal pain suggests ileocaecal disease, and lower abdominal pain suggests that the pain arises in the colon, renal tract or female internal genitalia.

The quality of the pain may also point to the cause. Pain in appendicitis, diverticulitis and pelvic disease is often described as aching. Cramping (colicky) pain suggests obstruction of a hollow viscus (small bowel, bile duct, ureter). A sensation of tearing, particularly radiating to the back, suggests aneurysmal dissection or rupture. A burning sensation suggests gastro-oesophageal reflux disease (GORD) or peptic ulcer disease.

Acute mesenteric ischaemia is often overlooked, even by experienced doctors. Severe pain out of proportion to physical signs, especially if atrial fibrillation is present, suggests acute mesenteric ischaemia. It is common for vomiting and/or evacuation of the bowels to occur at the start of the pain. The situation may progress rapidly to mesenteric infarction, which often proves fatal.

In an otherwise well patient, the longer is the history of abdominal pain, the less serious is the cause (this rule is not infallible). You should ask about factors that bring on/exacerbate the pain or alleviate the pain. Peptic ulcer disease, biliary disease and cancer are often related to food. Alleviation by antacids or other drugs that suppress gastric acid production (H_2 antagonists, proton pump inhibitors) is typical of peptic ulcer disease and GORD. Note that chronic mesenteric ischaemia is also commonly induced by eating (abdominal angina), and the patient may avoid food to prevent it (weight loss). Weight loss is also associated with underlying cancer, as is anaemia. Review medications: NSAIDs induce ulceration and a number of drugs may cause hepatic damage or pancreatitis (as does alcohol). Pain radiating to the back is associated with posterior abdominal structures (stomach, duodenum, pancreas, aorta). Previous abdominal surgery increases the likelihood of adhesions causing obstruction.

Examination of a patient with abdominal pain

Vital signs must be recorded (temperature, pulse rate and rhythm, blood pressure). Check for jaundice (biliary disease, liver disease and pancreatitis). Is there evidence of previous surgery? Bruising in the flanks or around the umbilicus suggests pancreatitis and a poor prognosis. Is the abdomen distended (obstruction, ascites)? Ask the patient to indicate where the pain is experienced and start light palpation away from that area and gently move towards it. After completing light palpation, feel the abdomen more deeply, searching for masses, enlarged abdominal organs and aneurysm. Are there any abdominal bruits? Guarding, rigidity, rebound tenderness and diminished bowel sounds suggest peritoneal inflammation, and a surgical referral will be needed. Distension of the abdomen with increased bowel sounds suggests intestinal obstruction. Do a rectal examination looking particularly for blood.

Peptic ulcer disease

This refers to both gastric and duodenal ulcers. NSAIDs are a major risk factor, but most patients will have infection with *Helicobacter pylori*. Only about 50% of patients have abdominal pain, and acute or chronic blood loss may be what suggests the diagnosis. The diagnostic test is upper GI tract endoscopy: any ulcers will be biopsied and samples will be sent to test for the presence of *H. pylori*. If an ulcer is suspected or demonstrated, NSAIDs should be withdrawn and treatment with a proton pump inhibitor (e.g. omeprazole) should be given for at least 8 weeks. If *H. pylori* is present, it can be eliminated by double antibiotic therapy (e.g. clarithromycin with metronidazole or amoxicillin). The gastroenterologist who did the endoscopy will usually give you instructions about this.

Sometimes, patients present with symptoms suggesting peptic ulcer disease but have normal investigations. This situation is referred to as non-ulcer dyspepsia. It is difficult to treat and you should get the advice of a gastroenterologist.

Gastro-oesophageal reflux disease

This is exceptionally common among older people. The classical complaint will be a retrosternal burning sensation, sometimes radiating to the mouth or throat. Sour-tasting fluid may be regurgitated. Sometimes, cough, wheezing or laryngitis may be the main complaint. Patients should undergo upper GI endoscopy. Ranitidine is usually effective at controlling symptoms. If it fails, a proton pump inhibitor should be used. Anti-reflux surgery is seldom recommended for older people, and endoscopic treatments remain unproven.

Ilioinguinal and genitofemoral neuralgias

Ilioinguinal neuralgia and genitofemoral neuralgia often go undiagnosed. Ilioinguinal neuralgia is caused by compression of the ilioinguinal nerve as it passes through the transversus abdominis muscle at the level of the anterior superior iliac spine. Genitofemoral neuralgia is caused by compression of the nerve as it arises from the L1 and L2 nerve roots, or of the genital/femoral branches as they pass beneath the inguinal ligament. L1 radiculopathy presents similarly. The pain is often burning or stabbing and there may be paraesthesiae over the lower abdomen, and sometimes radiating into the leg, scrotum or labia. The patient often assumes a bent-forward position when sitting. When lying, the knee is often held slightly flexed and internally rotated. Tapping the nerves often induces pain and paraesthesiae (Tinel's sign). The nerves may be damaged during unaccustomed and over-zealous activity, but, more commonly, by surgery (inguinal, hip or pelvic).

PAIN: BACK (SPINE)

Most back pain is not life-threatening or acutely disabling, but some causes are. To avoid overlooking one of these very serious problems, always examine the place that the patient experiences the pain. Ask the patient to localise the place with a finger. We have recently encountered a patient whose initial problem was pain in the upper thoracic spine which was initially treated symptomatically with analgesics. The patient deteriorated and on admission to hospital, had fever and a productive cough. He was treated as a case of community-acquired pneumonia (occasionally pain can be referred to the back). Nobody examined his thoracic spine until he developed signs of spinal cord compression. At surgery, a spinal epidural abscess was drained: the patient remains paraplegic. The Trust involved admitted negligence in failing to diagnose the abscess.

Lumbar spine

Most back pain is experienced in the lumbar spine and it is very common. The causes that are severe and serious are:

(1)   Cancer (primary and secondary);

(2)   Infection (osteomyelitis, abscess);

(3)   Fracture;

(4)   Pancreatitis;

(5)   Pancreatic cancer;

(6)   Gastric cancer;

(7)   Aortic aneurysm;

(8)   Peptic ulcer disease;

(9)   Pyelonephritis (flank).

Less urgent and benign causes include:

(1)   Degenerative joint disease;

(2)   Spondylolisthesis;

(3)   Spinal stenosis;

(4)   Disc herniation;

(5)   Muscle strain.

History

The first question to ask is whether the pain is confined to the back. If it radiates through the buttock and below the knee, a herniated disc or spinal stenosis should be suspected. Bilateral radiation down the legs suggests a central disk herniation (a neurosurgical emergency): there may be neurological signs attributable to the sacral nerve roots (saddle anaesthesia, bowel dysfunction, bladder dysfunction). Most degenerative disorders of the back improve with rest and worsen with activity: pain that persists unabated with rest, particularly when it disturbs sleep, suggests infection or cancer. Always check for any known diagnoses of cancer. Patients with lumbar spinal stenosis complain of leg pain with walking (especially downhill) or extension of the lumbar spine, heavy legs and back pain. This is sometimes confused with vascular claudication caused by arterial disease: vascular claudicants generally have worse pain going uphill while the opposite is usually the case for those with lumbar spinal stenosis. The pain of spinal stenosis is relieved by sitting or bending forwards.

Examination

Local swelling, redness and warmth suggest infection. Assess spinal movements: no limitation in spinal movements, or pain not exacerbated by spinal movement, increases the likelihood of an explanation that lies outside the spine. You need to do a detailed neurological examination of the legs and look for a sensory level (cord compression): if present, this is a neurosurgical emergency. You will also need to examine the abdomen and breasts.

Pain radiating down the leg with less than 60° of hip flexion on straight leg raising suggests irritation of the L4–L5 or L5–S1 nerve roots. Loss of the patellar tendon stretch reflex (knee jerk) suggests a lesion affecting the L3–L4 root. Unilateral loss of the Achilles tendon stretch reflex (ankle jerk) suggests an S1–S2 lesion: bilateral absence is common among older people. Decreased sensation over the medial calf and decreased dorsiflexion of the foot point to an L4 root lesion. Decreased sensation over the medial foot and decreased dorsiflexion of the big toe suggests an L5 root lesion. Decreased sensation over the lateral foot suggests an S1 root lesion. Reduced sensation in the posterior thigh and around the anus suggests lower sacral root lesions. Multiple root lesions or reduced sacral root sensation are indications for a spinal MRI scan: refer urgently for neurosurgical advice.

Fever or evidence of inflammation on blood tests suggests infection: refer for help. Weight loss and wasting is suggestive of cancer. Examine for enlarged lymph nodes and abdominal masses (cancer, aneurysm). In women, examine the breasts for lumps. In men, you need to do a rectal examination for possible prostate cancer.

Management

If there is a sensory level or any suggestion of cauda equina syndrome, refer urgently to a neurosurgeon. If cancer, fracture or infection is suspected, get plain radiographs and act according to the result. Evidence of cancer or aneurysm also indicates the need for further advice. Otherwise, treatment should be symptomatic. Prolonged bed rest (> 2–3 days) should be discouraged. Analgesia should be given using the principles we set out on page

151. The physiotherapist should introduce back exercises and mobilisation. If symptoms do not subside within 4–6 weeks, seek the advice of an orthopaedic surgeon.

PAIN: CALF

Calf pain is usually not symptomatic of serious disease. Possible causes are:

(1)   Muscle cramp;

(2)   Muscle injury (sprain, tear);

(3)   Referred from knee;

(4)   Cellulitis;

(5)   Peripheral vascular disease;

(6)   Radicular pain (L4–L5);

(7)   Deep vein thrombosis;

(8)   Neuropathy (usually alcohol or diabetes).

There are other rare causes that we have not listed.

Muscle cramp

Cramp is common among older people, especially night cramps. Cramp may be symptomatic of electrolyte disorders and, occasionally, of specific muscle disorders. Plantar flexion at the ankle may trigger cramp, and sleeping with an ankle–foot orthosis may prevent this. Otherwise, quinine sulphate is often given to variable effect.

Muscle injury

This usually occurs with unaccustomed exercise or injudicious movements. The pain comes on immediately with the injury and may be severe. Provided that the Achilles tendon has not ruptured (which is treated surgically), initial treatment is with rest and analgesics.

Cellulitis

This most often occurs on the forefoot in patients with diabetes and on the anterior or lateral leg otherwise, especially in patients with chronic oedema.

It is a circumscribed, spreading infection of the skin. It is discussed in more detail on page 183.

Peripheral vascular disease

This can cause pain acutely as a result of an embolus. It is particularly likely in those with atrial fibrillation. The pain may be very severe and there may also be paraesthesiae. Below the level of the embolus, the limb will be dusky and pulseless. It may feel cold. This is an emergency and salvage of the limb is by embolectomy, although occasional cases can be managed with anticoagulants. Embolectomy requires only local anaesthesia and is suitable for most patients. Failed embolectomy is managed by amputation or palliative care.

Chronic ischaemia is implied by claudication – pain induced by walking and which disappears on rest. Claudication may also be caused by lumbar spinal stenosis (page 163). Management is by life-style modification, control of risk factors for vascular disease and pain management. There are currently no drugs recommended for the specific management of peripheral vascular disease, although cilostazol appears to be a promising candidate. Severe vascular disease may induce rest pain. Functionally, patients are best served by retaining the limb, and treatment is focused on that. Reconstructive surgery should be undertaken, where possible. Patients requiring amputation of a leg will either require amputation of the other leg within 2 years or will have died. Amputee rehabilitation requires specialist input, often overseen by the local Disablement Services Centre.

Deep vein thrombosis

This presents with acute pain and tight swelling of the calf, or whole leg if the thrombus is more proximal. Immobility (stroke, heart failure), recent surgery (especially orthopaedic), obesity and cancer are the major risk factors. Those known to be at particular risk are given antiembolism stockings and low-dose heparin as prophylactic measures. On examination, the leg will be swollen and warm. The most serious complication is venous thromboembolism to the lungs. Take care not to misdiagnose cellulitis as a venous thrombosis.

The test most often used to aid diagnosis is the measurement of D-dimers. The test is not very specific for 'ruling-in', as many other conditions can raise D-dimer levels. However, a normal value is a very effective way to 'rule-out' the diagnosis. Duplex ultrasonography is the most often used imaging test to help in making the diagnosis, although the gold-standard remains contrast venography. Treatment is by full anticoagulation, initially with heparin and followed by warfarin (international normalised ratio (INR) kept between 2.0 and 3.0). The optimum duration of therapy is not known, but it is generally continued for 3–6 months after the first deep vein thrombosis (DVT). Recurrent DVTs are treated with lifelong therapy unless there are contraindications.

Neuropathy

In your practice, the most common neuropathies causing pain are those caused by diabetes or alcohol. Other features of the underlying disease will be apparent. There will be signs of sensory loss. Motor neuropathy will be suggested by clawing of the toes. Autonomic neuropathy will be suggested by a warm foot with dilated veins and other evidence of autonomic dysfunction. Treatment of the neuropathic pain is most often with antidepressants and/or gabapentin.

PAIN: CHEST

Chest pain is a common and potentially life-threatening problem, which must be taken seriously. The likely cause can often be determined on the basis of a history and physical examination without any further tests.

Commoner causes

(1)   Angina pectoris;

(2)   Myocardial infarction;

(3)   GORD;

(4)   Musculoskeletal pain;

(5)   Biliary colic;

(6)   Peptic ulcer;

(7)   Anxiety;

(8)   Shingles/post-herpetic neuralgia.

Rarer causes

(1)   Pulmonary infarct;

(2) Pericarditis;

(3) Rib fractures (trauma, coughing);

(4) Pneumothorax;

(5) Dissecting aneurysm.

The approach should be to rule out life-threatening causes before addressing more benign conditions. This means you should consider myocardial infarction, unstable angina, pneumonia, pulmonary embolism, pneumothorax and aortic dissection.

Very serious chest pain

History

Cardiac pain is usually described as pressure, heaviness or constriction which may radiate to the left neck and arm. It may sometimes be confused with pain arising from the oesophagus, although there will usually be other features of an oesophageal disorder (page 161). With stable angina, the pain is provoked by effort, and promptly responds to rest and nitrates. Unstable angina is provoked by lesser effort than before, lasts longer and may be slower to respond to rest and nitrates. The pain of myocardial infarction is persistent and not relieved by nitrates. Note that myocardial infarction can arise without pain. The pain of pulmonary embolism can be difficult to distinguish from ischaemic pain from the heart. Smaller pulmonary emboli may cause pleuritic pain (exacerbated by inspiration and coughing): similar pain may be seen in pneumonia, pneumothorax, aortic dissection and pericarditis. Pulmonary embolus and pneumothorax present with very-sudden-onset pain, often with associated breathlessness. Aortic dissection is also of sudden onset, is of a tearing nature and often radiates into the back. The pain associated with pneumonia is of more gradual onset and associated with cough, sputum and fever.

Co-morbid factors may point to the diagnosis. Vascular risk factors (pages 29, 79 and 128) and known aortic stenosis suggest ischaemic heart disease. Hypertension is the only known risk factor for aortic dissection. Chronic lung disease increases the likelihood of pneumothorax. Recent trauma/surgery, previous cancer and immobility increase the likelihood of pulmonary embolism.

Examination

Check the temperature, pulse and blood pressure. Rapid heart rate with hypotension suggests an acute coronary syndrome or pneumothorax. Hypertension suggests aortic dissection or a cardiac cause. The arm pulses may be asymmetrical with a dissecting aneurysm. A loud second heart sound suggests pulmonary embolism. An ejection murmur (radiating to the neck) points to aortic stenosis. Tachypnoea and low oxygen saturation suggests pulmonary embolism, pneumothorax or a coronary event with heart failure. The neck veins may be distended in pulmonary embolism, pneumothorax or a coronary syndrome. Reduced (or absent) breath sounds on one side of the chest suggest a pneumothorax: percuss the chest wall for hyper-resonance. Bibasal fine crackles suggest left ventricular failure. A friction rub may occur with pulmonary embolism or pericarditis.

Less serious chest pain

This may arise in the skin, muscles, costochondral joints, ribs or oesophagus. Pain may also be referred from the stomach, gall bladder or pancreas. Very early shingles or post-herpetic neuralgia may be described as burning or shooting: the skin over the affected area may be very tender to touch (allodynia). This may also arise after chest surgery. Rib fractures may arise after prolonged coughing or trauma: there will be localised tenderness at the fracture site. When traumatic, there is usually overlying bruising. Patients with costochondral syndrome often hold their shoulders in a fixed, neutral position: shrugging the shoulders and coughing reproduce the pain. Pain of a burning character suggests GORD.

Investigations and management

The most urgent investigations are an ECG and CXR. ST segment elevation on the ECG strongly suggests myocardial infarction (MI). If there are no Q waves, it is termed a 'threatened Q wave MI' as it frequently progresses to a 'Q wave MI' (full thickness MI). The enzyme creatine kinase rises soon after the onset of symptoms. A normal troponin T measurement more than 8 hours after the onset of symptoms makes a diagnosis of MI very unlikely. If MI is suspected, transfer the patient to the Heart Care Unit. Give intravenous opiates, oxygen and aspirin (chewed, not swallowed). Intravenous diuretics must be given if there are signs of pulmonary oedema. You may not feel confident to administer thrombolytic treatment, which must be given as soon as possible, and at least within 12 hours of symptom onset.

The local A&E department will have a protocol for this, so send the patient there as an emergency and warn them that you have done so if you have been unable to secure direct admission to the heart-care unit. Subsequently, β-adrenergic antagonists and ACEIs will be started.

Acute cardiac pain with ST depression and/or T wave inversion is also a medical emergency (which does not benefit from thrombolysis). Patients should be given oxygen, aspirin (chewed, not swallowed), a chewable nitrate, intravenous opioid (if the pain is ongoing) and subcutaneous low-molecular-weight heparin. They need urgent transfer to the acute medical service, where intravenous nitrates and β-adrenergic antagonists will probably be given in the heart-care unit.

If aortic dissection or pneumothorax is thought likely, send the patient urgently to the A&E department and warn them that you have done so. Patients suspected to have had a pulmonary embolus or pericarditis should also be transferred quickly to the acute medical service.

The other causes of pain do not require such urgent intervention, and it is wise to seek a medical opinion. Costochondral pain and rib fractures can be managed symptomatically with analgesics: NSAIDs are the most appropriate in the absence of contraindications. Patients known to have angina pectoris, whose pain resolves promptly with rest and sublingual nitrates, do not require referral unless they have recurrent, frequent episodes.

PAIN: EVERYWHERE

This is not a definable clinical syndrome, but is not an uncommon complaint in clinical practice. It implies axial pain, pain on both sides of the body and pain both above and below the waist. The pain may be localised to bone, joints and/or muscles, and is commonly associated with fatigue and stiffness. The complaint of 'pain everywhere' can be very challenging to diagnose, as the potential causes are many. Also, the severity of the underlying causes ranges from relatively minor to life-threatening. In your practice, depression will be a common underlying disorder but it may not be the cause: depression tends to make almost any pain worse, so you need to consider other possible causes (Table 4.5).

Approach to a patient with pain everywhere

A detailed history covering all body systems will be necessary because of the many potential causes. Pay particular attention to the onset of the symp-

Table 4.5 Possible causes of 'pain everywhere'

Drugs	Infection
Quinolone antibiotics	Viral (commonly)
Glucocorticoids	Bacterial (seldom)
Aciclovir	
Statins	Endocrine
Clofibrate	Hyperthyroidism
β-Adrenoreceptor antagonists	Hypothyroidism
Calcium channel blockers	Osteomalacia
Procainamide*	Glucocorticoid excess (may be
Hydralazine*	iatrogenic)
Isoniazid*	Hyperparathyroidism
Phenytoin*	Addison's disease
Tetracyclines*	
	Neuromuscular
Rheumatic	Myopathies
Fibromyalgia	Myositis
Myofascial pain syndrome	
Polymyalgia rheumatica	Cardiovascular
Polyarthropathy	Vasculitis
SLE	Endocarditis
Polymyositis/dermatomyositis	Atrial myxoma
	Psychiatric
Cancer	Depression
Widespread bony metastases	Somatisation disorder
Leukaemia	
Lymphoma	
Multiple myeloma	

*May cause drug-induced systemic lupus erythematosus (SLE)

toms, shorter histories tend to have more serious causes, although viral infections will generally present with a short history and fever. Ask about stiffness, which may point to disorders of the joints or muscles. Muscle cramps, muscle pain and muscle tenderness point to a primary muscle disorder or a condition that affects muscle (drug side-effect, metabolic disturbance). A past history of cancer should prompt you to consider the possibility of bone metastases. Go through the patient's medications one by one and check whether any of them has been associated with arthralgias, arthritis or myalgias.

A full physical examination is also needed. Fever points to inflammation (infection, inflammatory arthropathy, myositis). In your examination, pay particular attention to the joints (pain, swelling) and muscles (weakness, tenderness). Also examine carefully for enlarged lymph nodes.

The battery of screening tests we listed earlier in the book (page 5) will usually suffice. However, C-reactive protein (CRP) elevations will suggest an inflammatory cause. If there is any suggestion of a muscle disorder, check the creatine kinase (CK). Imaging procedures are not suitable as screening tools in this situation; consider them only if you have a definite question to answer.

If the likely cause is a medication, this should be withdrawn. Treatment of the pain with analgesics is appropriate while you are searching for an underlying cause. If there is depression, treat this too. If you have not made a diagnosis after assessing the patient and reviewing the investigations, refer the patient to a geriatrician.

PAIN: HAND AND WRIST

Pain in the hand(s) is a common complaint in old age. It can arise from any of the structures present in the hand: skin, tendon sheaths, synovium, bone and joints. The pain may be acute, intermittent or chronic. Most often, the pain will be caused by joint disease. Fortunately, the major causes of joint disease often have a characteristic distribution in the hand.

Joint disease

The major arthropathies affecting the hand in old age are:

(1)   Rheumatoid disease;

(2)   Osteoarthritis;

(3)   Gout;

(4)   Pseudo-gout (pyrophosphate crystal arthropathy).

Rheumatoid disease is a symmetrical, inflammatory polyarthropathy. When joints are involved in active rheumatoid disease there will be associated synovial thickening and soft tissue swelling. Osteoarthritis is a degenerative arthropathy which produces little by way of inflammation, and there is therefore little or no soft tissue swelling. Gout is an intensely inflammatory monoarthropathy caused by the deposition of uric acid crystals. Uric acid characteristically precipitates from solution in joints of low temperature (foot, hand) where its solubility is less than at core body temperature.

Entrapment neuropathies

The commonest is probably carpal tunnel syndrome, arising from compression of the median nerve, often bilaterally, as it passes under the flexor retinaculum. It is associated with rheumatoid disease, acromegaly, hypothyroidism, uraemia and amyloidosis. The pain classically affects the thumb, index, middle and radial half of the ring finger. A common complaint is waking owing to the pain. The sensory loss is over the ulnar border of the thumb, index, middle and radial half of the ring finger and extending to the wrist anteriorly, but only to the base of the affected fingers posteriorly. There is weakness in the abductor pollicis brevis, flexor pollicis longus, opponens pollicis and flexor digitorum profundus. The median nerve may also be trapped between the heads of the pronator teres muscle. The features are similar to carpal tunnel syndrome except that there is pain along the flexor side of the proximal forearm. The anterior interosseous nerve, a motor branch of the median nerve, may also be compressed over the interosseous membrane, but there is just hand weakness without pain. Pain is also a prominent feature of brachial plexopathy, but is never experienced in the hand alone.

Other causes of hand pain

A history of trauma will suggest a fracture: there will often be bruising and localised tenderness. Ganglion cysts are a common cause of wrist pain. Occasional patients will have hypertrophic osteoarthropathy, usually associated with a lung tumour. It affects the wrists most severely but may also affect the digits: finger clubbing will virtually always be present. Acute tendon sheath infections are very painful and associated with tenderness and swelling of a digit, which can come to appear sausage-shaped. De Quervain's tenosynovitis is an inflammatory tendon sheath disorder affecting the abductor pollicis longus and extensor pollicis brevis. It is attributed to 'overuse'. It causes pain and tenderness around the radial styloid process that is exacerbated by movement. Swelling is an uncommon associated finding.

Raynaud's syndrome, a vasospastic disorder associated with a number of connective-tissue diseases, can induce cold white hands, usually on cold exposure. Emboli to the upper limb can produce acute ischaemia with severe hand pain (the patient usually has atrial fibrillation, occasionally infective endocarditis).

Occasionally, especially in patients whose wrists have been restrained, and sometimes with diabetes, cheiralgia paraesthetica (handcuff neuropathy) develops. This is a compression neuropathy of the superficial dorsal sensory branch of the radial nerve (radial side of thumb and dorsoradial side of hand). Ulnar flexion of the hyperpronated forearm may reproduce the pain. The condition is usually self-limiting.

Approach to the patient with hand pain

While we have described a number of causes of pain in the hand, most patients will have a musculoskeletal disorder to explain it. Get the patient to show where the pain is experienced precisely. Look for evidence of swelling and deformity and feel for tenderness. Assess the range of movement and note any crepitus. Undertake a neurological examination of the hand, although sensory loss is unlikely in the absence of paraesthesiae and numbness. Assess muscle wasting and weakness and check the upper limb deep tendon reflexes.

The location of symptoms in the hand points to the likely cause:

(1)   Distal interphalangeal joints (osteoarthritis, psoriatic arthropathy, gout);

(2)   Proximal interphalangeal joints (osteoarthritis, rheumatoid disease, psoriatic arthropathy, systemic lupus erythematosus (SLE));

(3)   Metacarpophalangeal joints (rheumatoid disease, crystal arthropathy);

(4)   First carpometacarpal joint (osteoarthritis);

(5)   Wrist (rheumatoid disease, crystal arthropathy, ganglion cyst, carpal tunnel syndrome);

(6)   Radial styloid (De Quervain's tenosynovitis).

Management

Osteoarthritis, De Quervain's tenosynovitis and crystal arthropathy should be treated with simple analgesics. Active rheumatoid disease, SLE and Raynaud's patients should be referred to a rheumatologist. Entrapment neuropathies need to be confirmed by nerve conduction studies. A hand surgeon will be the most appropriate person to treat the entrapment.

PAIN: KNEE

There are a number of causes of pain in and around the knee:

(1)   Osteoarthritis;

(2)   Rheumatoid disease;

(3)   Infection;

(4)   Bursitis;

(5)   Ligament/tendon strain;

(6)   Ligament tear (cruciate ligaments);

(7)   Meniscus tear;

(8)   Tendinitis;

(9)   Fracture;

(10) Cancer (usually metastatic);

(11) Referred pain (radiculopathy).

Osteoarthritis

Osteoarthritis of the knee is by far the commonest cause of pain in the knee/distal femur. Chondromalacia patellae is osteoarthritis of the anterior compartment. Abnormal tracking of the patella on knee extension causes wearing of the anterior compartment cartilage. The pain is often worse when going upstairs or sitting. Otherwise, the pain of OA of the knee is felt diffusely. It is caused by movement and weight-bearing and is relieved by rest and, sometimes, local heat. Grating and popping sensations may be additional complaints. As the condition progresses, the range of movement at the joint diminishes and the knee becomes stiff. Often, there is evidence of wasting of the quadriceps femoris muscle in advanced osteoarthritis of the knee. The pain is generally sensed diffusely: localised pain should point you to a localised cause. Advanced osteoarthritis leads to deformity of the knee. You will seldom encounter a joint effusion. If the lower leg seems to deviate outwards from the knee, it is called genu valgus; it is very often bilateral.

Plain radiographs are usually diagnostic. Treatment is by analgesia (page 151), quadriceps strengthening and mobilisation. The most effective treatment for the pain is joint replacement. Patients whose pain fails to respond to the above measures should be referred to an orthopaedic surgeon.

Rheumatoid disease

This is a symmetrical, inflammatory arthritis of an autoimmune aetiology. The diagnosis will almost always have been made before you see the patient. The knee will seldom be affected alone. However, patients with rheumatoid disease have an increased vulnerability to septic arthritis, the signs of which may be suppressed by the immunosuppressive treatments used to control this disorder. If a single joint appears to be more troublesome than others, or develops swelling, you should get the opinion of a rheumatologist. The drugs you may encounter in patients with rheumatoid disease include:

(1)   Analgesics;

(2)   Glucocorticoids;

(3)   Sulphasalazine;

(4)   Methotrexate;

(5)   Azathioprine;

(6)   Gold salts;

(7)   Hydroxychloroquine;

(8)   Cyclosporin-A;

(9)   Infliximab.

Septic arthritis

This presents as pain in a patient who usually has additional features of infection such as fever and malaise. The patient will usually have a raised temperature. The joint will be swollen, warm and tender. The signs may be subtle in patients with rheumatoid disease owing to the use of disease-modifying drugs. There will be signs of joint effusion. Diagnosis is by joint aspiration (which will also differentiate it from crystal arthropathy). You need the urgent help of a rheumatologist or orthopaedic surgeon if you suspect septic arthritis.

Symptoms localised to part of the knee, clicking, locking, giving way

Pain or other symptoms that localise to part of the knee suggest localised causes such as ligament and tendon strains, meniscus tears and cruciate ligament ruptures. You are not expected to be able to diagnose these conditions and you should seek the advice of an orthopaedic surgeon.

PAIN: NECK

Pain in the neck must always be taken seriously, as some of the underlying disorders are very disabling. However, most neck pain is benign and improves with symptomatic treatments. The disorders that cause neck pain may be present with and without associated neurological findings.

Pain with neurological findings

(1)   Trauma;

(2)   Tumour (metastatic, rarely primary);

(3)   Disc disease;

(4)   Infection;

(5)   Rheumatoid disease;

(6)   Cervical spondylosis.

Pain without neurological findings

(1)   Meningeal irritation;

(2)   Fracture;

(3)   Sprain/strain;

(4)   Osteoarthritis;

(5)   Rheumatoid disease;

(6)   Cervical spondylosis;

(7)   Fibromyalgia.

History in patients with neck pain

Was the onset acute or insidious? Deceleration injury (whiplash) may cause neck strain, which usually resolves spontaneously. Is the pain persistent or intermittent? What happens during neck movements (vertical and horizontal)? Is there any pain, paraesthesiae or numbness in the arms? Is there any dysfunction in the legs? Is there evidence of any rheumatic existing disorder? Is there any evidence of a sensory level? Prolapsed intervertebral discs generally cause nocturnal awakenings owing to pain followed within hours to days by symptoms of a radiculopathy. Pain will usually be worse sitting or standing, and is relieved by lying down with the shoulder abducted. Valsalva's manoeuvre exacerbates the pain.

Chronic, nagging central cervical pain radiating to the occiput and sometimes to the shoulders, arms or chest is characteristic of cervical spondylosis. The degenerative changes are usually between C4 and C7. Pain is least troublesome on rising and worsens throughout the day. With canal stenosis, wasting of arm muscles, stiffness and walking problems develop. Dizziness may occur on neck movement. Giant osteophytes may cause dysphagia.

Examination of patients with neck pain

In the absence of direct acute trauma, you should assess the range of motion and the directions of movement that induce pain. This is usually done with the patient sitting. Is there any other evidence of rheumatoid disease? Is there spasm of the paraspinal muscles? Are there any trigger points? A screening neurological examination is indicated, paying particular attention to signs of cervical radiculopathy or cord compression.

If the leg deep tendon reflexes are exaggerated and there are upgoing plantar responses, spinal cord compression is likely. Reduced upper limb deep tendon reflexes or other features suggestive of a radiculopathy (pain in a dermatomal distribution) indicate that the problem is clearly in the cervical spine. Rheumatoid disease most often affects C1–C2 and osteoarthritis usually affects C4–C7. Look for a sensory level: it is often easier to ask the patient to do this with their own finger. A central lesion of the cord affects pain and temperature selectively in the arms. Rheumatoid disease usually causes cervical myelopathy by causing atlantoaxial subluxation. Osteoarthritis usually does so by the formation of bony spurs or ligamentous hypertrophy that impinges on the nerve roots.

Investigations and management

Most people you see will have chronic neck pain with no neurological findings. Generally, further investigation is not needed. Acute/recent onset of pain, a history of trauma or neurological symptoms and signs indicate that plain radiographs should be done. Patients with acute traumatic injuries should be assessed by the spinal surgeons or neurosurgeons: manage as we have described for head-injury patients needing transfer (page 121). All patients with evidence of disc prolapse, infection affecting the cervical spine or tumours must be transferred to the spinal surgeons or neurosurgeons.

The spine in cervical spondylosis is vulnerable to even minor trauma. The condition is generally managed with analgesics and physiotherapy if there are no neurological signs. Patients with neurological change should be considered for decompressive laminectomy.

PAIN: SHOULDER

Shoulder pain is very common, second only to back pain as a musculoskeletal problem: 20% of older people have complaints referable to the shoulders. In those with rheumatoid disease, there are shoulder complaints in about 80% of patients. The causes of shoulder pain include:

(1)   Joint (osteoarthritis, rheumatoid disease, septic arthritis, crystal arthropathy);

(2)   Surrounding tissues (rotator cuff tears, subacromial bursitis, bicipital tendinitis, suprascapular nerve entrapment);

(3)   Bone (fracture, dislocation, metastases);

(4)   Thoracic outlet syndrome;

(5)   Brachial plexopathy;

(6)   Referred (cervical spine, heart, gall bladder, diaphragm, liver, Pancoast's tumour);

(7)   Shoulder–hand syndrome (reflex sympathetic dystrophy);

(8)   Fibromyalgia.

Assessment and management

A history of trauma suggests fracture, dislocation or rotator cuff tear. Acute pain without trauma may arise from acute bursitis, tendinitis or rotator cuff dysfunction. Occasionally, crystal arthropathy or septic arthritis causes acute shoulder pain. Chronic shoulder pain is commonly caused by rheumatoid disease, osteoarthritis, rotator cuff dysfunction and fibromyalgia.

You need to test both the active and passive range of motion and find evidence of some more generalised arthritis. Subacromial bursitis causes localised tenderness at the acromion. Patients with rotator cuff dysfunction have normal flexion and extension. The first 15° of abduction can be achieved (deltoid), but usually not thereafter. If you passively abduct the arm to 90° and ask the patient to lower it slowly, with rotator cuff tears it drops (drop arm test). Plain radiographs of the shoulder usually give helpful diagnostic information.

Management depends on the cause. Suspected fractures, dislocations or septic arthritis should be referred to the orthopaedics and trauma service urgently. Active rheumatoid disease and crystal arthropathy should be referred to the rheumatologists. Suspected metastases, thoracic outlet syndrome and brachial plexopathy should prompt a referral to the geriatricians initially. Other patients should be given analgesics and physiotherapy. Rotator cuff tears that fail to improve can be treated surgically: minimally invasive surgery is becoming increasingly popular.

PALLIATIVE CARE

Palliative care developed as the needs of dying cancer patients who could not have curative treatment were recognised. Such care aims to promote quality of life with relief of symptoms in dying patients. The approach to care is holistic, and provides support to the patient and his/her family. Developed for the care of patients dying from cancer, the need for palliative care for patients with chronic diseases such as heart failure and COPD is increasingly recognised, but poorly provided. Specialist palliative care hospices for dementia patients exist in the USA but are not yet available in the UK. Whereas palliative care was once considered to be treatment *after* 'active treatment', it is now recognised that symptom control through palliative care treatment is often required *throughout* the course of a patient's illness and not just at the end of an illness.

In patients with advanced dementia, it is important to recognise that someone is dying. The terminal decline in incurable cancer is generally easily recognised: it is inexorably and fairly quickly progressive towards death. Conversely, terminal decline in the dementias (and many other chronic diseases) is generally slower, and is typically punctuated by abrupt declines in health (often caused by respiratory infections), which only partially recover, and during any one of which, the person may die. Fluids and antimicrobial chemotherapy may prevent death in one such episode, only for another episode to follow soon after. Thus, frequently recurrent acute illnesses in patients with advanced dementia, especially respiratory infections, are markers of the terminal decline of these patients, and active treatment interventions will generally be inappropriate and often quite ineffective. Similarly, feeding difficulties become increasingly frequent and problematic, with waxing and waning of the intake of food and fluids until no meaningful food or fluid intake becomes possible. There is now a general consensus that for most such patients, artificial fluids and hydration are not indicated, and, if given, will not affect the outcome in any meaningful or measurable way. These feeding difficulties too are symptomatic of the terminal decline. There is increasing use of care pathways to manage patients in the terminal phase of their illness, although none is available that specifically addresses the time course and nature of the problems associated with dying in advanced dementia.

Hospitalised patients can be referred to the palliative care team directly, who will either provide advice and expertise on the ward or arrange transfer to a palliative care unit. Discharge home for care can sometimes be supported. General practitioners can also refer to palliative care consultants and their teams or share care with specialist nurses experienced in providing terminal care at home.

RASHES

Skin diseases represent a gap in the knowledge and training of most doctors. If you do not recognise a skin rash, the chances are that a general physician or geriatrician will not recognise it either: you need a dermatologist's opinion. Nevertheless, some skin conditions are sufficiently common or sufficiently serious that you might be expected to know something about them. The conditions that we consider to fall within this group are:

(1)   Actinic keratoses;

(2)   Asteatotic dermatitis (xerosis);

(3)   Basal cell carcinoma;

(4)   Blistering diseases;

(5)   Cellulitis;

(6)   Contact dermatitis;

(7)   Drug eruption;

(8)   Intertrigo;

(9)   Leg ulcers;

(10) Melanoma;

(11) Pressure ulcers;

(12) Rosacea;

(13) Scabies;

(14) Seborrhoeic dermatitis;

(15) Senile purpura;

(16) Shingles;

(17) Squamous carcinoma;

(18) Stasis dermatitis (chronic venous insufficiency).

Actinic keratoses

Actinic keratoses are precursor lesions of squamous carcinoma. They tend to occur on the face, lips, ears, back of the hands and forearms (all sun-exposed). Characteristically the lesions are up to 1 cm in diameter, and appear as rough, gritty to the touch, adherent scaly white papules, often on an erythematous base. If actinic keratoses are suspected, the opinion of a dermatologist should be sought, not least because the condition is effectively and simply treated.

Asteatotic dermatitis

This occurs in dry, usually itchy, skin. In this setting, reticular erythematous patches, scales, fissures and slightly raised plaques may occur, often on extensor surfaces of the arms and the anterior tibial skin. The scaling is because corneocytes are shed in clumps, rather than singly. Sometimes the scaling and fissures resemble crazy-paving (eczema craquélé).

It is always associated with dry skin, and treatment is aimed at reducing water loss in recently hydrated (after bathing) skin using moisturisers and emollients (occlusive moisturisers). Soap used during bathing should be mild or oilated. Vaseline® is effective at maintaining skin hydration but it is often not very acceptable to patients. Oils and emulsifying ointment (ung. emulsificans) may be added to bath water, though they tend to make the bathtub slippery. The BNF lists numerous emollients.

Basal cell carcinoma

These occur most often on the sun-exposed parts of the head and neck and preferentially in areas with many sebaceous glands (e.g. naso-labial furrow). They are usually (but not always) raised, nodular and pearly with prominent telangiectasis. The centre often ulcerates and crusts. They are locally invasive but rarely metastasise. Treatment is usually straightforward and effective: refer the patient to a dermatologist.

Blistering diseases

Small blisters (< 5 mm diameter) are called vesicles, and larger ones are called bullae. Blisters may be a feature of pressure ulceration, and they occasionally complicate diabetes mellitus and venous stasis in the legs. The most commonly encountered blisters in geriatric practice arise during an episode of shingles (see later). All other causes of (usually large) blisters are serious, and the opinion of a dermatologist must be sought urgently. The situation is particularly urgent if the emergence of blisters follows starting a new drug or during/after an infection (possible toxic epidermal necrolysis/Stevens–Johnson syndrome).

Cellulitis

Cellulitis is a localised spreading infection of the skin and is characterised by redness, swelling, pain and fever. There is generally a clear edge to the redness and swelling, and red, tender lymphatic vessels may be seen extending from it. Cellulitis is commonest on the legs, particularly in the setting of chronic oedema. The most likely organisms are streptococci and staphylococci. 'Blind' antibiotic treatment with penicillin and flucloxacillin is appropriate.

Rarely, the seriousness of the situation may be underestimated, and the true diagnosis may be necrotising fasciitis. Consider this in a patient who is extremely ill or in whom pain in the affected part seems out of proportion to the observable clinical findings. Necrotising fasciitis is limb- and life-threatening: treatment must not be delayed. The definitive treatment is radical surgical debridement and antibiotics. If necrotising fasciitis seems possible, get the advice of a surgeon.

Contact dermatitis

The rash is usually (but not always) localised to the area of contact with the cause. Common causes are substances present in jewellery, hair products, skin products, cosmetics, latex and antibiotic-containing ointments. The rash is usually intensely itchy. Acutely, it may comprise vesicles and erythematous and/or oedematous plaques. These may erode, revealing exudate with crusting. Chronically, the plaques may become lichenified and pigmented. Scabies and irritant dermatitis may have a similar appearance. If the area affected remains localised, treatment is with topical glucocorticoids, and a more generalised rash is treated with systemic glucocorticoids. If this condition is suspected, refer to a dermatologist. The offending cause must be avoided.

Drug eruption

Morbilliform eruptions

The commonest form of drug eruption is described as morbilliform (measles-like). It is thought to be a type-II hypersensitivity reaction. It arises up to 8 weeks after starting the offending drug and is occasionally fatal. The drugs most often implicated include penicillins, sulphonamides, NSAIDs, anticonvulsants and antihypertensives. The patient may be febrile. The rash is generally symmetrical on the upper body and comprises erythematous macules and papules. Confluent areas may be seen. The rash is usually not itchy. Similar rashes may be seen with viral illnesses and collagen vascular diseases. Internal organs may also be involved (lymph nodes, liver, kidney). Treatment is by withdrawal of the offending drug and topical or systemic glucocorticoids.

Urticarial eruptions

Urticarial eruptions are the second commonest, representing type-I hypersensitivity. In a patient already sensitised, the rash may arise within minutes of administering the drug. Cutaneous erythematous wheals are seen. Subcutaneous involvement is called angioedema and may affect the larynx and/or the bronchial tree. In addition, anaphylactic shock may occur.

Fixed drug eruptions

Fixed drug eruptions occur as one or a few erythematous patches. For unknown reasons, the genitalia and perianal areas are favoured sites for fixed drug eruptions. Patients may complain of pain, itching and burning at the site of the rash. The rash may blister (bullous fixed drug eruption) or form crusts. The lesions typically heal with pigmentation. Sulphonamides, tetracyclines and NSAIDs are the commonest causes.

Photosensitivity

The rash resembles sunburn and typically affects the face, hands and upper chest: shaded areas (under chin) and covered areas are spared. In severe cases, blisters may form.

Lichenoid drug eruptions

These are rare. The name comes from the resemblance to lichen planus. Typically, purple, scaling papules occur which are itchy and are commonly distributed on the trunk and extremities. They may be exudative and form crusts. It may progress to an exfoliative dermatitis. Gold, captopril, calcium channel antagonists and β-adrenergic antagonists are the commonest causes.

Erythema multiforme

This is a rare form of drug eruption which can also arise in mycoplasma and herpes virus infections. It typically presents with target-shaped lesions arising from concentric rings of erythema and pallor. Lesions can be macular, papular, urticarial or vesicular (bullous erythema multiforme). Often, the lesions are first seen on the palms and soles, but the rash becomes widespread and occasionally affects mucosal surfaces. Very severe erythema multiforme affecting skin and mucous membranes is called Stevens–Johnson syndrome: this is life-threatening.

Intertrigo

This is superficial inflammation at areas of skin apposition where there is frictional trauma, warmth and moisture. There may be mixed, localised infection with yeasts and skin bacteria. The commonest sites affected are:

(1)   Below the breasts;

(2)   Groin;

(3)   Between abdominal fat folds;

(4)   Intergluteal cleft;

(5)   Axilla;

(6)   Umbilicus.

The earliest change is blanching erythema in a 'kissing' (where the skin surfaces oppose) pattern that progresses to a subacute dermatitis with weeping and sometimes crusting. There may be fissuring at the depths of the fold. It occurs more commonly in people with diabetes or those taking antibiotics. Urinary or faecal contamination may exacerbate the dermatitis.

Treatment is by washing with mild soap, rinsing thoroughly and trying to maintain aeration. If severe, wet dressings (2% acetic acid, potassium permanganate: one Permitabs® in 4 litres of water) for 30 minutes four times a day for 2–3 days can be very effective. Do not do this for more than this period, as secondary changes attributable to the wet dressings may occur. After the wet dressing and patting dry, apply Timodine® or Canesten® cream. Continue to apply the cream for at least 14 days after the wet dressings have stopped. These creams can be used for longer periods as prophylaxis against recurrence. If there is extensive superficial infection, use silver sulphadiazine cream for the first 2 weeks. If the measures just described do not bring about marked improvement within a week, seek the advice of a dermatologist.

Leg ulcers

There are many causes of leg ulcers, but in your practice, the commonest causes are:

(1)   Venous ulcers;

(2)   Arterial ulcers;

(3)   Vasculitic ulcers (associated with rheumatoid disease).

The treatment of leg ulcers will depend on the underlying diagnosis. Venous ulcers arise as a result of venous hypertension. The sign of chronic venous hypertension is shiny, non-pitting, brawny oedema. There is usually brownish pigmentation (haemosiderin). Not all patients with venous hypertension develop ulcers. Those who do often do so recurrently. The most effective treatment is compression using triple-layer bandaging. The tissue viability nurse (TVN) will be skilled at this. Otherwise, the vascular surgery service may need to be involved.

An absolute contraindication to compression is the presence of significant peripheral vascular disease: the TVN will screen for this by calculating the ankle/brachial pressure index (ABPI). Peripheral vascular disease and venous hypertension may coexist. Arterial ulcers can be induced to heal in some circumstances: these patients need to see a vascular surgeon.

Vasculitic ulcers are most often seen in patients with rheumatoid disease. The diagnosis can be confirmed by skin biopsy. Treatment is with glucocorticoids. All other ulcers need specialist knowledge for diagnosis: ask a dermatologist or geriatrician.

Pressure ulcers

These occur at sites of tissue compression against a non-compliant surface for longer than the tissues can tolerate. The early features suggest that ischaemia–reperfusion is a critical phenomenon in their development. The earliest stage is blanching erythema of the skin, which gives way to non-blanching erythema, superficial ulceration and, then, deep ulceration. The ulcers may extend sufficiently deep to expose muscle, tendon and bone. Prevention is better than cure, and your nurses should be assessing pressure ulcer risk and taking appropriate action. The commonest sites at which they develop are:

(1) Sacrum (lying);

(2) Trochanters (lying);

(3) Ischial (sitting);

(4) Heels (lying, footstool).

Treatment is by relief of pressure, debridement and dressings to promote the removal of devitalised tissue and support wound healing. In some countries, more extensive use is made of plastic surgeons to close pressure ulcers using flap rotation. You need specialist advice for the adequate management of pressure ulcers and you should approach the TVN or geriatrician.

Rosacea

This most often develops between the ages of 40 and 50 years but can arise in old age. Also, the effects of untreated rosacea will persist into old age. The earliest features are flushing of the face and nose. Erythematous papules develop on the nose, cheeks, forehead and chin. Telangiectasis and further erythema may develop. The nose may become bulbous (rhynophyma), and blepharitis and conjunctivitis may occur. Treatment is by using sunscreens and antibiotics. The antibiotics may be applied topically or be given systemically (e.g. doxycycline, 100 mg twice daily)

Scabies

This is caused by the mite, *Sarcoptes scabei*, which inhabits burrows in the stratum corneum of the skin, where eggs are laid. The commonest places to find them are the interdigital webs of the hands, ventral wrist and the shaft of the penis. Spread is by person to person contact, and you will be at risk of acquiring scabies yourself. You should look carefully for ridges, about 1 cm long with a dark dot at one end (the mite). Not only does the mite lay eggs in the burrows, but it also deposits faeces. The host responds with immune-mediated inflammation. Later changes include papules, nodules, eczematous dermatitis, crusted plaques (Norwegian scabies) and, sometimes, vesicles and bullae (bullous scabies). Usually, a host is colonised by only a small number of mites, but in Norwegian scabies, there can be thousands of them.

If the burrows can be identified or you have a strong suspicion that the diagnosis is scabies rather than atopic dermatitis, contact dermatitis or drug eruption, the best plan is to treat with topical malathion or permethrin. Treatment is often recommended for close contacts and household members. Norwegian scabies may benefit from simultaneous oral treatment with ivermectin (available only on a named-patient basis).

Seborrhoeic dermatitis

The lesions are erythematous patches and plaques which appear oily, and frequently form scales. The lesions characteristically appear between the eyebrows and nasolabial folds, on the scalp and, sometimes, on the chest. It is sometimes mistaken for rosacea. It is associated with overgrowth of a commensal yeast, *Malassezia furfur*. Treatment is with ketaconazole cream and shampoo.

Senile purpura

This appears as bruises at sites subjected to recurrent minor trauma, especially the backs of the hands and forearms. The bruises often fail to go red and take a very long time to clear. They are associated with thinning of the skin. The walls of capillaries may also be thinned and predispose them to rupture. Extravasated blood spreads easily in the thin skin, where there are fewer macrophages to remove it. The underlying changes are generally attributed to aging changes. Similar changes occur in people on treatment with glucocorticoids for long periods of time. No investigation or treatment is needed.

Shingles (zoster)

This is caused by the varicella zoster virus, which also causes chicken-pox. After the initial infection, the virus is not completely eliminated, but remains dormant in dorsal root ganglia. Reactivation of the virus can happen for no obvious reason or in association with some other acute illness or immunosuppression.

Tingling and pain arise in the affected dermatome, followed hours later by a rash. The rash first appears as papules which progress to form blisters. The blisters subsequently ulcerate. This is usually followed by healing as the immune response clears the virus. Sometimes, especially in the immune-suppressed, systemic infection resembling chicken-pox occurs.

When the vesicles form blisters, the patient becomes infective to others and remains so until healing occurs within 3–4 weeks. Scars may remain after healing. Patients need to be isolated from those who have not had chicken-pox or received the vaccine. Treatment is by antiviral treatment, usually aciclovir orally. This must be given within 48–72 hours of the rash appearing. This treatment reduces acute pain, accelerates healing and reduces the risk of post-herpetic neuralgia. Aciclovir is given intravenously in disseminated zoster. It is also known that the incidence of post-herpetic neuralgia is reduced by treating with a tricyclic antidepressant or an anti-convulsant from the start until healing has occurred.

Squamous carcinoma

This is a malignant tumour that arises from keratinocytes above the basal layer of the epidermis. Ultraviolet light exposure is the major risk factor, and it often develops from actinic keratoses. In its earliest form, it appears as a firm papule, often scaly. As the lesion enlarges, central ulceration is the rule. It may also bleed. If you suspect a squamous carcinoma, you should feel the regional lymph nodes and refer urgently to a dermatologist. Early treatment, increasingly using Moh's surgery, produces excellent results.

RECTAL BLEEDING

Rectal bleeding is a common problem in elderly patients. Causes range from minor local conditions to life-threatening blood loss. Occasionally, massive upper GI bleeding with rapid gut transit can present as a fresh rectal bleed.

Rectum and anus

(1)   Haemorrhoids;

(2)   Anal fissure.

Colon

(1)   Diverticular disease;

(2)   Angiodysplasia;

(3)   Cancer;

(4)   Inflammatory bowel disease – ulcerative colitis and Crohn's disease;

(5)   Ischaemic colitis.

Clinical features

Bleeding from haemorrhoids and anal fissures is typically associated with constipation. Bright-red bleeding is noticed on toilet paper or in the toilet bowl. Perineal pain may be experienced with anal fissures or strangulated haemorrhoids.

Bleeding with colonic cancer is usually seen as blood mixed with stool, and there may be a history of change in bowel habit. Abdominal pain may be experienced.

The presence of blood clots usually indicates bleeding above the haemorrhoid-bearing level. Bleeding in inflammatory bowel disease is usually associated with diarrhoea and the passage of mucus.

Diverticular bleeding is typically associated with large rectal bleeds. Angiodysplasia may present similarly. An acutely ill patient with sudden onset of severe abdominal pain, shock and bloody diarrhoea is a typical presentation of acute ischaemic colitis.

Management

The patient should be assessed for the severity of the bleeding. Pulse and blood pressure should be checked. Tachycardia, systolic hypotension, postural hypotension or an episode of loss of consciousness suggest significant blood loss. Good venous access should be obtained and initial volume replacement should begin with a plasma expander such as gelofusin. Blood should be taken for cross-matching, full blood count, urea and electrolytes and clotting. The surgical team should be contacted as an emergency, and arrangements for transfer made after the patient is stabilised.

Management of milder bleeding is less urgent. Abdominal examination may reveal a mass. A rectal examination should be performed (page 56). Anal fissures may be observed as a crack or triangular ulcer at the anal verge. Haemorrhoids may be visible. Tumours in the rectum or anal canal may be palpable as a hard ulcer crater. Patients with rectal bleeding are usually referred to the surgical team for further assessment, which might include sigmoidoscopy, barium enema examination or colonoscopy.

STROKE

Stroke is the third commonest cause of death after ischaemic heart disease and cancer. Up to one-third of patients die within a year of a stroke, and half of the survivors are left dependent. Stroke medicine is a rapidly developing area, and strong evidence-based guidelines on the provision of services and management of strokes have been produced.

A stroke is defined as the clinical syndrome of rapid onset of a focal or global cerebral deficit lasting more than 24 hours or leading to death, with no apparent cause other than a vascular one. A transient ischaemic attack (TIA) is defined similarly with resolution of symptoms within 24 hours. When patients are seen within 24 hours of symptom onset, good clinical practice is to regard all as having an emergency 'brain attack', akin to 'heart attack', which may or may not recover in hours, days or weeks.

Ischaemic stroke accounts for 80% of strokes, primary intracerebral haemorrhage 15%, and 5% are due to subarachnoid haemorrhage. Other causes of strokes are rare, particularly in older patients. Half of all ischaemic strokes are due to atherothrombotic disease of the extracranial arteries, one-fifth are due to cardiac emboli and about a quarter are due to lacunar infarcts – occlusion of small, deep, perforating cerebral arteries. The risk factor most closely related to stroke is hypertension. Atrial fibrillation is the most important risk factor for embolic stroke. Other vascular risk factors include diabetes, smoking and obesity. Stroke incidence rises with age. Pre-existing vascular disease such as ischaemic heart disease or peripheral vascular disease is also associated with an increased stroke risk, as is heart failure. The relationship between stroke and plasma cholesterol is less straightforward, although treatment with statins in patients with vascular disease does appear to reduce stroke incidence.

Sudden-onset hemiparesis, hemisensory disturbance, hemianopia and dysphasia are typical stroke presentations. Strokes in the vertebrobasilar territory may present with cerebellar signs, cranial nerve palsies and hemi- or quadriparesis. Stroke symptoms are typically negative phenomena. TIAs usually present with transient loss of speech, weakness or loss of vision in one eye (amaurosis fugax). Examination of suspected strokes should include assessment of heart rhythm, blood pressure, listening for heart murmurs, examination of the chest for evidence of aspiration pneumonia and a full neurological examination. Check the temporal arteries for swelling and tenderness. Swallowing should be assessed, but if in doubt about the safety of swallowing keep the patient 'nil by mouth' and commence intravenous fluids. Investigations should include full blood count, urea and electrolytes, blood sugar (BM stix is essential if consciousness is disturbed, to exclude hypoglycaemia), ECG and chest radiograph. Patients should be commenced on aspirin 300 mg per day by mouth or per rectum.

Management

All suspected stroke patients should be referred to the medical team on-call. Most will require transfer to a medical unit, ideally a specialised stroke unit. Patients with TIAs usually recover well within 24 hours and may be managed on an out-patient basis, but all cases should be discussed with the medical team on-call.

Further management would include CT brain scanning to determine the type of stroke. Care centres on the avoidance of complications of stroke such as pressure ulceration, DVT and aspiration, whilst proceeding with rehabilitation. Further management assesses risk factors for stroke and the provision of secondary prevention treatment.

SWALLOWING PROBLEMS

Problems with swallowing are usually referred to as dysphagia. When there is painful swallowing, the term odynophagia is often used. Mechanical problems obstructing the passage of the contents of the buccal cavity and motility disorders of the oesophagus generally cause greater problems for solids than for liquids. When the underlying problem is neurological rather than mechanical/dysmotility, the difficulty is generally greater for liquids, which may also pass into the nose and induce coughing and spluttering on attempted swallowing. Neurological causes of swallowing problems may arise acutely (stroke, botulism) or subacutely (neurodegenerative conditions). In these patients, dyspraxias and agnosias may be underlying causes of swallowing problems.

Physiology of swallowing

The process of swallowing has been shown to occur in four stages:

(1) Oral preparation phase (in which food or liquid – the bolus – is chewed or manipulated in preparation for swallowing);

(2) Oral propulsive phase (in which the tongue pushes the food or liquid to the back of the mouth, beginning the swallowing response);

(3) Pharyngeal phase (in which food or liquid quickly passes through the pharynx into the oesophagus);

(4) Oesophageal phase (in which the food or liquid moves through the oesophagus into the stomach).

The first two stages are controlled voluntarily (cortical swallowing centres), while the latter two occur reflexly. The process involves rapid, precise coordination of numerous muscles and tissues of the mouth, pharynx, larynx and oesophagus. When the bolus (food or fluid) enters the pharynx, the soft palate elevates to close off the nasopharynx and the hyoid bone and larynx move upwards and forwards. The vocal folds move to the midline and the epiglottis folds backwards, protecting the airway; the effect of the epiglottis is small. The tongue pushes backwards and downwards into the pharynx, thereby moving the bolus down. The pharyngeal walls assist this process by moving inwards with a progressive wave of contractions from top to bottom. The upper oesophageal sphincter relaxes and is pulled open by movement of the hyoid bone and larynx (used as a sign in the bedside assessment of swallowing), and then the sphincter closes after the food passes. Once in the oesophagus, a peristaltic wave moves the food downwards. The lower oesophageal sphincter relaxes and allows the bolus to move into the stomach. After the food is in the stomach, this lower sphincter closes to prevent reflux of gastric contents. Contrary to popular belief, the presence or absence of a gag reflex has no relationship to someone's ability or inability to swallow safely.

Investigation of swallowing problems

If food sticks, try to ascertain the level of sticking. Take a detailed history of the nature of the problem. Try to get a witness description, particularly in patients with dementia. In essence, you are trying to differentiate a mechanical cause of dysphagia from a neurological one. Try to observe the patient swallowing water and feel the larynx during the swallow. Observe for coughing or spluttering. Always examine the mouth for local problems that may impede adequate chewing. Perform a screening neurological examination paying special attention to the cranial nerves.

If the cause is thought to be mechanical, a barium or gastrografin swallow is usually the first-line investigation as it identifies not only any mechanical obstruction, but also disorders of motility. If an obstruction is found, an endoscopy is usually done to determine whether it is a benign or malignant obstruction. Endoscopy is also used in the treatment of both benign and malignant strictures (dilatation, stents).

In patients with neurological causes of swallowing problems, a clinical assessment is usually done at the bedside to assess the safety of the swallow. It is wise to ask a speech and language therapist to undertake this assessment. Subsequent investigation may be by videofluoroscopy, during which the entire process of swallowing can be observed in detail. Increasingly in the USA, direct observation of the larynx and pharynx using endoscopy and foods/liquids of different consistencies and containing a green dye is being done (flexible endoscopic evaluation of swallowing with sensory testing; FEESST). This procedure is quicker, and may give additional information.

Recognising feeding problems in dementia

Patients with dementia may have feeding problems for many reasons. They may forget to eat, may not recognise food, may be distracted during eating, may have problems chewing and initiating swallowing and may fail to coordinate swallowing and protect the airway. The nurses/carers will often be aware of a number of problems:

(1)   Being unaware of food when it is presented;

(2)   Holding food in the mouth;

(3)   Difficulty chewing;

(4)   Difficulty moving food to the back of the mouth;

(5)   Spitting food out;

(6)   Eating very quickly;

(7)   Putting too much food into the mouth;

(8)   Refusing food and/or drink;

(9)   Talking with food or drink in the mouth and forgetting to swallow;

(10) Coughing/choking on food and/or fluids;

(11) Complaints of food not going down or getting stuck in the throat;

(12) A 'wet' or 'gurgly' voice after swallowing;

(13) Difficulty swallowing tablets.

Treatment of swallowing problems

Mechanical disorders may be treated endoscopically or surgically. Motility disorders are treated medically. In many stroke patients, the swallowing problems improve/resolve. Occasionally, when there are problems with elevation of the larynx, laryngeal suspension surgery can be done. This is seldom curative but it may help. If the swallowing problem persists, food and nutrition may need to be given through a feeding tube, though this may increase the likelihood of respiratory infections. In patients with advanced dementia and other progressive neurological disorders, particularly in their late stages, this sort of intervention is usually not very effective. Before considering it, other strategies should be attempted.

Making feeding safer

Positioning

(1)   Sit upright at a 90° angle;

(2)   Tilt head slightly forwards;

(3)   Remain sitting upright or standing for 15–20 minutes after eating a meal.

Dining environment

(1)   Minimise distractions in the eating area;

(2)   Remain focused on eating and drinking;

(3)   Do not talk with food in the mouth.

Amount and rate

(1)   Eat slowly;

(2)   Cut food into small pieces and chew it thoroughly;

(3)   Eat small amounts per swallow.

Swallowing

(1)   Swallow two or three times per bite or sip;

(2)   Cough gently or clear the throat after each swallow, and swallow again before taking a breath.

Saliva management

(1)   Drink plenty of fluids;

(2)   Periodically suck on ice chips or drink lemon-flavoured water to increase saliva production.

Food consistency

(1)   Eat soft foods;

(2)   Puree food;

(3)   Thicken liquids.

Taking medications

(1)   Crush tablets and mix them with pudding;

(2)   Consider liquid formulations of drugs.

TREMOR/MOVEMENT DISORDERS

A tremor is an involuntary, rhythmic movement across a joint. It may be present at rest (*resting tremor*), on posture (*postural tremor*) or on movement (*kinetic tremor*). *Chorea* is an irregular, arrhythmic, unpredictable brief movement involving the extremities in a continuous, random order. *Athetosis* is a slow, writhing, more proximal movement. When there are features of both chorea and athetosis, the term *choreoathetosis* is used. *Myoclonus* is a series of brief, shock-like contractions of one or more muscles which cause movements across a joint. *Tics* are rapid, brief, repetitive, stereotyped movement, commonly affecting the face or axial muscles. *Dystonia* is a sustained muscle contraction which may cause abnormal postures. *Fasciculations* are brief twitches in a group of muscle fibres and indicate denervation. *Clonus* is a rhythmic movement precipitated by sudden stretching of a tendon. It is most often seen at the ankle. Clonus indicates an upper motor neurone lesion and is usually associated with very brisk deep tendon reflexes. *Akathisia* is a sense of restlessness and a feeling of the need to move. *Restless legs syndrome* refers to intense discomfort in the legs and an intense desire to move them.

Many patients are aware of the abnormal movement, and may therefore seek to incorporate it into some seemingly purposeful movement. There are many types of tremor and movement disorder. We describe here only those that we feel are particularly relevant. More detailed information can be found in a neurology textbook.

History

Many movement disorders are familial, so take a family history. Alcohol is associated with alleviation of essential tremor but may cause a cerebellar tremor. Always take an alcohol history. Take a drug history too. Also note any associated medical conditions.

Examination

Undertake a screening neurological examination including an assessment of gait. The finger–nose test is abnormal in cerebellar hemisphere disease, sensory impairment and essential tremor. Examine the handwriting of the patient and get him/her to draw a spiral.

Observe whether the movement disorder is present at rest, on posture or on movement. Is tone normal, increased or decreased? Are the deep tendon reflexes normal, increased or decreased? Is the patient's posture normal or abnormal? Is the head involved and is there any incoordination?

Parkinsonism

Parkinson's disease is a degeneration affecting the substantia nigra which is responsive to L-dopa and other dopamine agonists. As well as the tremor, there is gait abnormality, akinesia and rigidity. Other disorders can cause Parkinsonism and these do not respond to L-dopa. Common causes include phenothiazines, butyrophenones, Lewy body disease, diffuse cerebrovascular disease, multisystem atrophy, progressive supranuclear palsy, olivopontocerebellar atrophy, traumatic encephalopathy and carbon monoxide poisoning. Referral to someone with an interest in movement disorders is indicated unless it is clearly related to neuroleptic drugs.

The tremor is characteristically a rest tremor of the hands and fingers. It is often referred to as pill-rolling. It is absent during sleep and declines on posture and movement.

Essential tremor

This is a coarse tremor which may be present at rest and is worsened by posture and movement. It may affect the hands and head, but rarely the legs. Alcohol may markedly suppress it. When this tremor develops in old age, it is often called senile tremor. The rest of the neurological examination is normal. It sometimes responds to long-acting β-adrenergic antagonists. Gabapentin and topiramate have sometimes been used to treat essential tremor.

Neuroleptic drugs

Akathisia can develop soon after starting neuroleptics (and sometimes, metoclopramide, antihistamines or paroxetine) and may be mistaken as agitation, which precipitates the prescription of more neuroleptics. Patients with akathisia often go on to develop tardive dyskinesia. This most commonly manifests as sustained, rhythmic movements of the tongue and mouth, lip-smacking and facial grimacing. Neuroleptics may also induce dystonic reactions, especially retrocollis and partial opisthotonos, which may persist after drug withdrawal.

Tetrabenazine, anticholinergics and botulinum toxin have been used to treat dystonia. The best treatment of tardive dyskinesia is to avoid neuroleptics. β-adrenergic antagonists, anticholinergics, benzodiazepines and clonidine may suppress akathisia.

Primary orthostatic tremor

This is a lower limb-tremor induced by standing, and disappears on sitting and walking. Patients often say it feels like 'jelly' when standing still. When you observe the patient, the knees appear to be shaking. Auscultation over the lower-limb muscles often sounds like the rotor blades of a helicopter. If this is suspected, request an electromyogram (EMG). The tremor may ameliorate with L-dopa, clonazepam or primidone, but not with β-adrenergic antagonists or alcohol.

Cerebellar tremor

This is noted only on movement. It indicates cerebellar hemisphere abnormalities and it may be bilateral. In the finger–nose test, the tremor worsens as the finger nears its target. It is associated with impaired alternating movements and hypotonia. Speech may be abnormal: it is called scanning speech and sounds rather like a 'Dalek'.

Huntington's chorea

This is a dominantly inherited disorder that rarely presents in old age. Early features are clumsy movements, slow movements and a tendency to drop things. Eventually, dementia develops. Psychosis may arise, and depression with suicide attempts is not unusual. The abnormal movements are jerky, often associated with slower dystonic movements. The abnormal movements can be exacerbated by sustained actions such as fist clenching or tongue protrusion.

Dystonia

This is a sustained, abnormal posture, either focal or generalised. Focal dystonias may be task-specific (e.g. writer's cramp). The commonest dystonia is spasmodic torticollis, in which there is persistent contraction of the neck muscles. Dystonia is common in patients with Parkinson's disease taking dopamine agonists.

WEIGHT LOSS (UNINTENTIONAL) AND WASTING

Weight loss

Energy requirements decline in old age, and reduced food intake is a consequence. Resting energy expenditure is reduced, which reflects the reduction in lean body mass with advancing age. Reduced physical activity also leads to a reduced food intake.

A high proportion of elderly people are underweight, and inadeqate nutrition is a particular problem in hospitalised and institutionalised elderly subjects. Social, psychological and medical factors can all lead to weight loss. Treatable causes of weight loss should be identified. Depression should be sought and treated. Unnecessary dietary restrictions should be removed, and any appetite-suppressing drugs should be discontinued.

A dietary history should be taken to assess whether food intake is adequate. In hospitalised patients, food intake can be monitored by food charts, and response to dietary supplementation can be assessed by regular weighing. Oral food supplementation may suffice for some patients, but feeding via nasogastric tube (less than 6 weeks) or tube enterostomy (percutaneous endoscopic gastrostomy, PEG) for more long-term feeding may be required. There is little evidence for the benefit of appetite stimulants. Dietitians are helpful in advising on appropriate supplements and monitoring response. They will usually advise when response to oral supplementation is inadequate or intake remains poor, and suggest nasogastric tube or PEG feeding. The appropriateness of more invasive feeding supplementation should be determined in light of the individual's underlying diagnosis and potential for recovery.

Weight loss is a frequent indication for referral of elderly patients to medical out-patient clinics. Diseases in many systems can lead to weight loss, and review of the systems part of the medical history may pick up potential sources which will then guide investigations. Smoking history and alcohol intake should be determined. In smokers, a history of persistent cough or haemoptysis should be sought, possibly indicating a lung neoplasm. Upper gastrointestinal symptoms such as dysphagia, vomiting or epigastric pain should be sought and might indicate oesophageal or gastric cancer. Persistent diarrhoea might indicate malabsorption. A change in bowel habit or rectal bleeding may occur in colonic carcinoma. Thirst and polyuria might indicate diabetes mellitus. Heat intolerance, tremor and irritability may indicate hyperthyroidism. Clinical examination would include looking for signs of anaemia, finger clubbing and lymphadenopathy. In women, breast examination should be performed. Features of hyperthyroidism should be sought. Clinical signs suggesting underlying lung malignancy such as collapse or pleural effusion may be found. Abdominal examination is performed for palpable masses and hepatomegaly. Rectal examination should be performed to find tumours and to assess the prostate gland in men.

Clinical symptoms are used to guide investigations. However, the following blood tests are routinely performed: full blood count (FBC) to look for anaemia; urea and electrolytes are checked to indicate chronic renal disease; blood glucose should be measured to diagnose diabetes mellitus. Liver function tests might indicate liver metastases or alcoholic liver disease. Thyroid function testing is performed to diagnose hyperthyroidism. A bone profile may reveal a raised calcium or raised alkaline phosphatase level, which might indicate metastatic bone disease. A chest X-ray should be performed for all patients to look for primary or secondary lung neoplasms. Urine should be tested for haematuria. When baseline investigations do not indicate a likely cause of weight loss and weight loss continues, further tests are required. Gastrointestinal disease is the most likely cause. Gastroscopy, flexible sigmoidoscopy and barium enema examination are performed to identify the more common gastrointestinal causes of weight loss. The order of investigation is determined by symptoms, but sometimes no clinical indicators are present and all tests are required. An abdominal ultrasound scan to identify disease in the liver, kidneys and pancreas is also useful in unexplained weight loss. This test can be performed earlier in the order of investigation if there is hepatomegaly or abnormal liver function. Further investigations might include CT scans of the chest and abdomen.

For patients in whom weight loss persists and in whom no identifiable underlying cause is found, or in whom identified medical conditions have been treated, the prognosis is usually poor and nutritional interventions are not usually successful.

Reduced food intake is a feature of aging which reflects the reduction in basal metabolic rate. This is determined by lean body mass, which declines with age. Reduced physical activity also leads to a reduced food intake. A high proportion of elderly people are underweight, and inadeqate nutrition is a particular problem in hospitalised and institutionalised elderly subjects. Social, psychological and medical factors can lead to weight loss. Treatable causes of weight loss should be identified. Causes include:

(1) Depression;

(2) Dementia;

(3)   Visual impairment;

(4)   Neglect/elder abuse;

(5)   Alcoholism;

(6)   Monotonous diet;

(7)   Thyrotoxicosis;

(8)   Uncontrolled diabetes mellitus;

(9)   Malabsorption;

(10) Medications (digoxin, SSRIs, NSAIDs, anticonvulsants, antibiotics);

(11) Painful oral conditions;

(12) Xerostomia (dry mouth);

(13) Ill-fitting dentures;

(14) Swallowing disorders;

(15) Oesophageal obstruction;

(16) Peptic ulcer disease;

(17) Mesenteric ischaemia;

(18) Cancer;

(19) Chronic inflammatory disorders (rheumatoid disease, inflammatory bowel disease);

(20) Chronic infections (tuberculosis, autoimmune deficiency syndrome);

(21) Heart failure;

(22) COPD.

This list is by no means exhaustive.

Conditions that cause weight loss/wasting cover almost all body systems, so a full history and examination are required. A detailed history of eating and life-style is also needed. Unless there are specific features uncovered (e.g. chronic diarrhoea, steatorrhoea), the screening investigations we suggest should be sufficient. Measurement of C-reactive protein may point to an active inflammatory disorder. In your practice, depression and dementia will be common causes, but you should also consider that there may be other causes too. In particular, evaluate the drug chart for drugs that may induce anorexia or nausea. If the cause is still not clear, get the help of a geriatrician.

Treatment will focus on the underlying cause. In addition, unnecessary dietary restrictions should be removed and appetite-suppressing drugs discontinued. Recommend appealing foods, particularly those with high energy content (fat). Also, introduce high-energy food supplements such as Maxijul®. Food intake can be monitored by food charts, and response to dietary supplementation can be assessed by regular weighing. Oral food supplementation may suffice for some patients, but feeding via nasogastric tube (less than 6 weeks) or tube enterostomy for more long-term feeding may be required. There is little evidence for the benefit of appetite stimulants.

A person with depression complains of weight loss and tiredness

Depression would be the most likely diagnosis in someone with weight loss and prominent tiredness, for physicians as well as psychiatrists. When weight loss is reported, it is important to obtain objective evidence with serial weighing. Weight gain as depression improves is reassuring.

Tiredness is a common symptom, and is usually not due to a medical cause in over 90% of cases presenting to general practitioners. In a medical history, the patient's life-style would be assessed, their sleep pattern assessed and the impact of the symptom on function would be determined.

Weight loss too is a non-specific symptom, but is often due to serious illness. Diseases in many systems can lead to weight loss, and review of the systems part of the medical history may pick up potential sources which would then guide investigations. Smoking history and alcohol intake should be determined. The patient's diet should be assessed. In smokers, a history of persistent cough or haemoptysis would be sought, possibly indicating a lung neoplasm. Upper gastrointestinal symptoms such as dysphagia, vomiting or epigastric pain should be sought, and might indicate oesophageal or gastric cancer. Persistent diarrhoea might indicate malabsorption. A change in bowel habit or rectal bleeding may occur in colonic carcinoma. Thirst and polyuria might indicate diabetes mellitus. Heat intolerance, tremor and irritability may indicate hyperthyroidism. Clinical examination would include looking for signs of anaemia, finger clubbing and lymphadenopathy, features of hyperthyroidism and breast lumps in women. Signs of lung malignancy such as collapse or pleural effusion would be sought. Abdominal examination is performed for palpable masses and hepatomegaly. Rectal examination should be performed to look for tumours and to assess the prostate gland in men.

Clinical symptoms are used to guide investigations. However, the following blood tests are routinely performed: full blood count (FBC) to look for anaemia; urea and electrolytes would be checked to indicate chronic renal disease; blood glucose for diabetes mellitus. Liver function tests might indicate liver metastases or alcoholic liver disease. Thyroid function testing is performed to diagnose hyperthyroidism. A bone profile may reveal raised calcium or raised alkaline phosphatase, which might indicate metastatic bone disease. A chest X-ray would be performed for all patients to look for primary or secondary lung neoplasms. Urine would be tested for haematuria. When baseline investigations do not indicate a likely cause of weight loss and weight loss continues, further tests are required. Gastrointestinal disease is the most likely cause. Gastroscopy, flexible sigmoidoscopy and barium enema examination would be performed to identify the more common gastrointestinal causes of weight loss. The order of investigation would be determined by symptoms, but sometimes no clinical indicators are present and all tests are required. An abdominal ultrasound scan to identify disease in the liver, kidneys and pancreas is also useful in unexplained weight loss. This test would be performed earlier in the order of investigation if there was hepatomegaly or abnormal liver function.

An in-patient suddenly complains of abdominal pain

There are many causes of abdominal pain. Features that should be elicited are the site, time and nature of onset, severity, nature (burning, colicky, stabbing, etc.), progression of the pain, how it ends, duration, aggravating and relieving factors, radiation and any precipitating factors.

The site of the pain is most useful. Pain in the upper abdomen may be from the biliary tree, stomach and duodenum and the pancreas. Gallbladder pain may radiate to the shoulder tip, and stomach, duodenal and pancreatic pain radiate through to the back.

Pain in the central abdominal area arises from the small bowel and caecum plus the aorta. Pain from the kidney is felt in the lateral abdomen and the loin and may radiate to the groin.

Pain in the lower abdomen can arise from the appendix and caecum (right iliac fossa), bladder, uterus, ovaries and Fallopian tubes (hypogastrium) and the colon (left iliac fossa).

The character of the pain also gives clues to its origin. Abdominal pain can be divided into two broad categories. Pain due to inflammation is generally constant, and does not go away until the inflammation resolves. The pain is aggravated by pressure or change in tension of the peritoneum, such as occurs during palpation or movement. Pain may also occur where there is obstruction to a muscular viscus (bowel, ureter), and produces colic. This is a pain that fluctuates in intensity and is griping in nature. More rarely, abdominal pain may occur secondary to vascular disturbance such as arterial occlusion or rupture of an aneurysm. Pain is usually acute in onset and felt in the central abdomen. Radiation to the back may occur, and the onset is typically acute and severe. Pain in the abdomen may also be referred from other sites such as the spine, heart or lungs/pleura.

Associated symptoms may also help to localise the cause of pain. Nausea and vomiting tend to occur with upper gastrointestinal causes of pain. Altered bowel habit and absence of passing flatus and vomiting may indicate bowel obstruction. Dysuria and frequency point to urinary infection; inability to pass urine may indicate urinary retention. Vaginal discharge/bleeding may indicate pelvic infection or malignancy.

Any abdominal condition may occur whilst patients are hospitalised, but some problems occur more commonly. Constipation may produce griping abdominal pain in the left iliac fossa. Patients are usually extremely accurate in their recall of days without a bowel action, at least in the UK! Urinary infection may produce hypogastric discomfort, but should be accompanied by urinary frequency and dysuria. Diverticular disease is more common in the elderly, and may present with acute diverticulitis. Patients may be febrile with left iliac fossa pain and tenderness and a palpable mass. Sigmoid volvulus is also more common in the elderly. This usually occurs in a constipated individual who may present with sudden-onset severe colicky abdominal pain and rapid abdominal distension. A characteristic abdominal X-ray finding of a dilated single bowel loop resembling a coffee-bean may be seen. Colonic pseudo-obstruction is also more common. It is seen in patients with serious coexisting illnesses and with anticholinergic and psychotropic medication. Presentation occurs with abdominal distension but no features of absolute constipation. True obstruction should be excluded.

Patients with abdominal pain require careful and gentle examination. This is more likely to elicit important signs. Patients often appear to be in pain, and their position in bed and respiratory pattern may provide supportive evidence. Temperature, pulse and blood pressure should be measured. The abdomen should be inspected, and gentle examination made for tenderness and guarding, indicating peritoneal inflammation, and the presence of masses. The external genitalia and hernial orifices should also be examined. A rectal examination should be performed. A distended abdomen with increased bowel sounds may indicate intestinal obstruction.

Laboratory investigations rarely establish a diagnosis but are supportive. Routine tests would usually include FBC, urea and electrolytes, amylase if epigastric pain and vomiting is present and urinalysis for evidence of infection. C-reactive protein (CRP) is usually raised in infective or inflammatory processes. Plain abdominal radiographs are not generally helpful unless intestinal obstruction is present. If renal colic is suspected, a plain abdominal film may reveal renal stones. An erect chest radiograph may show free gas under the diaphragm when perforation occurs.

A patient with an acute pain in the abdomen will usually appear unwell. However, in the elderly these features may be attenuated, and diagnosis of acute conditions can be difficult. Advice from surgical colleagues will frequently be needed. After excluding simple problems such as constipation and urinary infection it is best to seek advice on further management.

A physically well woman attending the memory clinic has an ESR of 80

The erythrocyte sedimentation rate (ESR) is a non-specific test, and we do not recommend its use as a screening test. It is widely used for monitoring inflammatory or infective processes. The ESR rises with advancing age, which makes it less useful in older patients. ESR also rises in anaemia. Levels are raised in infection, inflammatory processes such as connective-tissue disease and malignancy. It is frequently performed as a speculative test, and if raised, poses the question – 'is there something going on?'

Unfortunately, the ESR is frequently raised in asymptomatic healthy patients. It is a poor screening test in healthy elderly people as it usually leads to a battery of further investigations which are frequently negative or do not point to a treatable diagnosis. Even worse, an orphan investigation results in the search for further diagnosis. This begs the question – why have you done the test? And the more difficult one to answer – can you ignore it?

Measuring the ESR in the elderly is useful in patients with suspected temporal arteritis. In patients with bone pain or anaemia in whom myeloma is suspected, a raised ESR is supportive, and it is also useful in monitoring treatment responses in inflammatory conditions.

Having obtained a high ESR result, it is necessary to ask questions about conditions that may produce it. Symptoms suggestive of malignancy such as weight loss, cough and haemoptysis, dysphagia, change in bowel, haematuria, etc. should be sought. Joint pain and stiffness may indicate inflammatory arthritis. Headache, scalp pain and jaw claudication may indicate temporal arteritis. Chronic infection may produce night sweats.

A full examination is required. Investigations will be guided by symptoms and clinical findings. A chest radiograph and a myeloma screen (protein electrophoresis and urine for Bence-Jones protein) are usually requested. Unfortunately, benign monoclonal gammopathy is common in the elderly, and may produce an abnormal electrophoresis result. Benign monoclonal gammopathy does not progress to myeloma. A skeletal survey and bone marrow aspiration may then be required to exclude multiple myeloma. These tests are usually negative, and the patient has had a sequence of investigations and a potentially alarming diagnosis, all for the sake of a pointless investigation. The bottom line is: never do an ESR unless you have a specific diagnosis in mind.

A routine chest X-ray in an in-patient prior to electroconvulsive therapy (ECT) shows a shadow at the left apex. There is a history of tuberculosis and she has smoked 20 cigarettes a day for 20 years

The differential diagnosis here is between reactivation of previous tuberculosis or a lung neoplasm. The radiologist's report should indicate the likely diagnosis. If a report is not available, the film should be discussed with a radiologist. Often, old radiographs are available for comparison, and may show no change, thus offering reassurance. Radiologists will usually recommend a CT scan of the chest if a neoplasm is suspected. Referral to a chest physician will be required. If reactivation of TB is suspected and the patient is producing sputum, it should be sent for staining and culture for TB. Tuberculin skin testing in the elderly is of little diagnostic value. The presence of 'open' tuberculosis (the patient is producing infected sputum) is a health risk to others, and the patient may require isolation in a side-room. Such a patient would be best transferred to a chest ward.

An elderly man with dementia in a nursing home has a rectal carcinoma which is inoperable and he is in great pain

Rectal pain in this situation can be a difficult problem to treat. The management of this patient's pain will to some extent be determined by what previous treatments have been given. The patient should be known to a surgical team and perhaps to the palliative care team. Pain treatment relies on the patient's description of the pain experienced. However, this patient may not be able to provide a description of his pain. Pain may occur solely on defaecation. For those patients experiencing pain on defaecation it is important to avoid constipation. Faecal softening or osmotic laxatives should be prescribed. Sometimes local, non-curative surgery helps.

Spasmodic or searing pain may be experienced, and a constant feeling of fullness is frequently described. Neuropathic pain from nerve root involvement and bony pain from tumour invasion of the sacrum may also arise. Several approaches should be considered.

Radiotherapy Pelvic radiotherapy can relieve pain and should be considered if not used previously and the patient is able to cooperate.

Analgesics Strong opiates will usually be required to relieve pain. Non-steroidal anti-inflammatory drugs (NSAIDs) may help if there is bony pain.

Adjuvant treatments Corticosteroids may be tried to help nerve root compression symptoms. Tricyclic antidepressants are used to treat neuropathic pain: anticonvulsants may also be used (see page 156).

Anaesthetic techniques A variety of nerve block techniques have been described to relieve rectal pain.

The best guidance for treatment of rectal pain in the case described will be from the palliative care team. The palliative care consultant will generally liaise with surgical, radiotherapy and anaesthesia colleagues to determine the most appropriate treatment.

A woman who has rheumatoid arthritis and depression is in pain

The treatment approach to this patient's pain will depend on several issues. First, is there active rheumatoid arthritis? Active rheumatoid arthritis is usually treated with disease-modifying anti-rheumatic drugs (DMARDs), which slow the rate of joint damage. Symptoms suggestive of active disease include morning stiffness (for over 1 hour), weakness, anorexia and weight loss and fatigue. There may be symmetrical pain, and swelling and tenderness of joints especially in the hands, wrists, knees and hips. The ESR is usually raised as are acute-phase proteins such as CRP, which reflect disease activity. Commonly used DMARDs include sulfazalazine and methotrexate, but many new treatments have become available recently. Patients with suspected active disease should be referred to a rheumatologist.

Non-steroidal anti-inflammatory drugs (NSAIDs) are used to relieve pain and inflammation but have no effect on disease activity. Side-effects in the elderly are common, including gastric irritation and gastrointestinal bleeding, renal failure and salt and water retention, which can aggravate hypertension and heart failure. Co-prescription with selective serotonin re-uptake inhibitors (SSRIs) may further increase bleeding risk. Newer agents which inhibit COX-2 enzymes (coxibs) have a lower incidence of gastrointestinal toxicity, but similar other side-effects. Recent concerns have been raised about the risk of myocardial infarction with coxibs. Traditional NSAIDs can be co-prescribed with proton pump inhibitors or misoprostol to provide gastric protection

In patients who have had rheumatoid arthritis, joint damage can ensue, with the development of secondary osteoarthritis. There may be little active inflammation in joints and pain is due to osteoarthritis. Simple analgesia with paracetamol either alone or combined with weak opioids can provide effective pain relief. Where one joint is especially painful, a steroid injection into the joint may provide pain relief. It is essential where one joint is inflamed to consider and exclude septic arthritis, and hospital admission for joint aspiration and culture may be required.

An 80-year-old lady admitted with dehydration and confusion refuses surgery for intestinal obstruction

It is quite common to see an elderly patient who refuses to have treatment. In a confused patient the dilemma is whether this represents a pre-held view or is a consequence of the confusional state. In this scenario it is essential that the diagnosis is correct. If surgery is thought to be possibly necessary, then it is worth involving the surgical team early. Not infrequently, surgeons are unwilling to operate on some elderly patients if they think the operative risks are too high. If this is the case, then much upset may be spared. Patients may also be able to make a better choice with the clear explanation of risks from a surgeon.

If surgery is feasible then the key issue is to determine whether the patient is making a competent decision. There are recognised components in determining competence which should be followed. If it is felt that the patient is making a competent decision, then their view should be respected. If relatives are contactable, then their view should be sought. If the patient has written an advance directive, then this too should be examined for guidance. Consensus between nursing, medical and surgical staff is reassuring in this situation. Having followed these steps, if surgery is believed to be a life-saving option and which may lead to resolution of the confusional state, then surgery should proceed. Appropriate assent forms are available, which are signed by two doctors, allowing surgery to proceed. For a detailed account of consent to medical treatment in Scotland, *see* Chapter 2, page 22.

A 78-year-old lady with an 18-year history of Parkinson's disease presents with severe restriction of mobility and a 2-year history of increasingly disturbing auditory and visual hallucinations. How might you manage her psychiatric symptoms without further impairing her physical function?

Psychosis as a feature of Parkinson's disease is usually drug-induced, and occurs most often as visual hallucinations in clear consciousness. The lifetime prevalence is about 50%, but the incidence increases with severity and duration of the disease. Patients with a history of cognitive impairment, increased age, history of depression or sleep disorder and daytime somnolence are most at risk. The majority of patients have no premorbid psychiatric disorder.

Dopaminergic drugs vary in their tendency to produce hallucinations due to their various binding characteristics at different dopamine receptors, but the 5HT (5-hydroxytryptamine) receptors in the cortex and limbic systems are also involved.

Hallucinations with preserved insight is *not* psychosis. The impact of psychosis in the Parkinson's patient is an increased risk of behavioural disturbances, higher mortality, a more rapid progression of motor symptoms and an increase in the rate of institutionalisation.

It is important when prescribing any anti-parkinsonian medication that patients and families are made aware of the possible side-effects. Any possible external triggers, e.g. infection, must be excluded as possible causes of a confusional state. Before considering the use of antipsychotic medication, some manipulation of the Parkinson medication should be attempted. These should be discontinued in the following order: anticholinergics; monoamine oxidase (MAO)-B inhibitors, e.g. selegiline; catechol-*O*-methyltransferase (COMT) inhibitors, e.g. pergolide; dopamine agonists, e.g. bromocriptine.

If these measures are ineffective or the patient is not receiving any of these treatments, then the L-dopa therapy must be reviewed. Ideally, a reduction in the overall daily dose should be the aim, starting with a decrease initially in the nocturnal dose. Continued small reductions in the daily dose should be continued until either the psychosis settles or the patient's mobility begins to decline. At all times, assessment of the physical state should be made, subjectively, or by the use of a rating scale.

When no further reduction in the L-dopa can be made without significant decline in function, the introduction of a small dose of antipsychotic must be considered. All antipsychotics carry some risk of exacerbating parkinsonian symptoms. The atypical antipsychotics carry the least risk, with a propensity to develop extrapyramidal side-effects in the order: risperidone > olanzapine > quetiapine > clozapine. Due to its complex monitoring and risk of blood dyscrasias, clozapine is rarely used. A small dose of quetiapine, e.g. 25 mg, may therefore be helpful as an alternative. Aripiprazole has reportedly no more risk of producing extrapyramidal symptoms than placebo, and may prove to be beneficial. It acts as a dopamine system stabiliser, agonistic in dopamine-depleted systems, and antagonistic in systems where dopamine is produced in excess. The starting dose can be as low as 5 mg daily.

The aim of therapeutic manipulation is to minimise psychiatric morbidity, whilst retaining or maximising physical function. A delicate balancing act often ensues, and some compromise of function may have to take place.

6   Commonly prescribed drugs

PRINCIPLES OF PRESCRIBING

Prescribing in the elderly

Older people are the greatest consumers of prescription medication, and are also frequent users of over-the-counter medications (OTCs). They are more likely to experience adverse drug reactions, and as multiple drug users are at risk of the effects of drug interactions. Multiple drug use is also more likely to lead to poorer compliance. Adverse drug reactions are an important cause of hospital admission in the elderly. For example, falls and their consequent injuries can occur as side-effects of psychotropic or vasoactive medication.

Older people are more sensitive to drugs acting on the central nervous system. Sedation and confusion are more likely to occur with opiates and benzodiazepines. The elderly are more likely to experience bleeding from non-steroidal anti-inflammatory drugs (NSAIDs) and aspirin, and they are more likely to experience a serious or fatal outcome as a consequence.

The response to drugs may differ in older people due to the effect of aging on pharmacokinetics and pharmacodynamics and/or the effect of accumulated diseases. Pharmacokinetic changes in drug absorption, distribution and metabolic clearance by the liver and kidneys are described. Reduced renal clearance makes an elderly person more susceptible to nephrotoxic drugs. Pharmacodynamic changes such as increased sensitivity to warfarin and reduced sensitivity to beta-blockers are reported.

Guidelines for good prescribing

Most of the following guidelines apply to all prescribing, but are particularly important for elderly patients:

(1) Always review the entire medication regimen of the patient whenever you see him or her.

(2) Aim to simplify prescription regimes to improve compliance.

(3) Discontinue any drug whose indication for use is no longer clear.

(4)   Start with a low dose and increase as needed slowly.

(5)   Always consider the potential for side-effects and their impact on the patient.

(6)   Always look for adverse drug effects and always consider the possibility of an adverse drug reaction as the cause of symptoms.

(7)   When selecting a drug from a particular class, try to choose a drug best suited to that particular patient.

(8)   Remember the potential interaction of any new medication with existing medications.

It is well established that inappropriate and excessive prescribing is extremely common for older people. More than 80% of older people take at least one medication daily. The drug trials that provide us with much of our information have often excluded old people. This is particularly so for women, who account for around 70% of our workload. Even when they have been included, those participating will have been highly selected and will not have been taking multiple other drugs, which may well interact with the drug(s) under study. Better information for practical purposes has generally come from pharmacoepidemiological studies (NSAIDs, benzodiazepines, hypoglycaemics). In the future, more such information will hopefully accrue. However, at present, the best information we generally have comes from clinical experience and inferences from what we know about age-related changes in pharmacokinetics and pharmacodynamics.

Pharmacokinetics

This refers to the absorption, distribution, metabolism and elimination of drugs. Although there have been many age-related changes described that may alter drug absorption, it turns out that the absorption of most drugs is relatively unaffected during aging.

Drugs distribute into the intracellular and extracellular spaces, and many age-related changes affect this. In particular, changes in body composition exert the following effects:

(1)   Reduced total body water;

(2)   Decreased albumin;

(3)   Increased fat–lean ratio.

Non-polar drugs that distribute in the body fat mass (e.g. diazepam) have a larger volume of distribution, whereas polar ones (digoxin, amino-glycosides, gabapentin) will have a reduced one. Low albumin levels, which are common in ill, older people, will have greater concentrations of free drug if the drug is significantly protein-bound. Also, drugs can compete for binding sites, so adding a new drug that is highly protein-bound (thyroxine, warfarin, digoxin) can displace other drugs (e.g. most anticonvulsants) and cause drug toxicity.

Drug metabolism varies between individuals and changes during aging. Drugs such as propranolol, which undergo high first-pass metabolism as they enter the liver, can be markedly affected by this. The major systems for drug metabolism are called phase I (oxidation, reduction) and phase II (conjugation). Phase II reactions do not alter significantly during aging but many phase I reactions decline. Renal excretion will depend largely on the glomerular filtration rate, which declines variably during aging.

Pharmacodynamics

This refers to how drugs exert their effects at the various tissue sites. Pharmacodynamic changes with age have not been well studied. However, many drugs given to older people may have unpredictable and paradoxical effects, which may arise from pharmacodynamic changes. This is especially true of all psychoactive drugs.

Adverse reactions to drugs

These occur more commonly in older people, particularly in those taking several drugs. Those taking five or more drugs will almost inevitably have an adverse drug reaction (ADR). ADRs account for a large number of hospital admissions. This is why you should always review the drug chart and check in the British National Formulary (BNF) when a patient develops a new problem, particularly if a new drug has been started. The name usually given to the co-prescription of multiple drugs is polypharmacy.

Risk versus benefit

Some drugs are so likely to cause unwanted effects that outweigh any benefit that they should rarely be prescribed for older people. These include sedating antihistamines, long half-life benzodiazepines and long-acting sulphonylureas.

Compliance

Compliance becomes increasingly difficult with multiple medications, and non-compliance occurs with 40–75% of older people. It is important to be aware of non-compliance, as doses may be inappropriately increased if the expected effect has not occurred. Sometimes, the non-compliance is highly desirable when it is prompted by ADRs and unwanted effects (intelligent non-compliance).

Better prescribing

Not all of life's ills should be treated with medications. When you see an older patient, make a conscious effort to reduce the number of prescribed drugs to the minimum needed. Never start a drug unless you are able to set a goal that you expect to be achieved. Also, set a time when you will review whether or not the goal has been achieved. If it has not, review the diagnosis, the goal and the prescribed drug.

When you start a drug, it is usually (but not always) wise to 'start low and go slow': start with a low dose and increase the dose at longer intervals than you would for younger people. Patients should be encouraged to report any new problems that arise after starting the drug.

Nobody can be expected to know all the details of all the drugs they encounter. Our best advice is to become confident with a small number of drugs and to use those preferentially. Any deviation from this 'personal pharmacopoeia' should prompt the prescriber to look up the drug in the BNF. For convenience, we summarise below the important details of many of the drugs commonly encountered in geriatric practice.

CARDIOVASCULAR/CEREBROVASCULAR DISEASE

Aspirin (acetylsalicylic acid)

Indications

This is indicated for the prevention of cerebrovascular events or myocardial infarction.

Side-effects/cautions

It should be used with caution in people with asthma, uncontrolled hypertension and peptic ulceration. Bronchospasm and gastrointestinal haemorrhage (other haemorrhages such as subconjunctival haemorrhage may occur) are the main side-effects. Enteric-coated aspirin (Nu-Seals® aspirin) is available.

Dosage   75 mg per day.

Clopidogrel

Indications

This is indicated for the prevention of ischaemic events in patients with a history of ischaemic disease, and, in combination with low-dose aspirin, is licensed for the treatment of acute coronary syndrome without ECG evidence of ST segment elevation (can be used as an alternative to aspirin).

Side-effects/cautions

It should be started in hospital in-patients only. It should be avoided for the first few days after myocardial infarction, and for 7 days after stroke, and in people with increased risk of bleeding. Discontinue 7 days before elective surgery unless an antiplatelet effect is specifically required.

Dosage   75 mg per day.

Dipyridamole

Indications

This is used as an adjunct to oral anticoagulation for the prophylaxis of thromboembolism associated with prosthetic heart valves, with modified-release preparations licensed for secondary prevention of ischaemic stroke. It can be used in combination with low-dose aspirin but long-term benefits have not been established. An available modified-release preparation is Persantin® Retard, and in combination with aspirin is Asasantin® Retard.

Side-effects/cautions

It should be used with caution in severe angina, recent myocardial infarction, hypotension and heart failure and may exacerbate migraine. Side-effects are mainly gastrointestinal, with dizziness, myalgia, throbbing headache and hypersensitivity reactions as well as increased bleeding.

Dosage   300–600 mg per day in 3–4 divided doses before food.

Diuretics

Generally, in older people, lower doses of diuretics should be used as the elderly are particularly prone to side-effects. Renal function should be measured and doses modified according to this. Simple gravitational oedema should not be treated long-term with diuretics, and support stockings and raising of the legs should be used as an alternative. Hypokalaemia is a particularly severe side-effect.

Thiazide diuretics (bendroflumethiazide)

These are moderately potent diuretics acting by inhibiting sodium reabsorption at the beginning of the distal convoluted tubule.

Indications

These include oedema and hypertension. In primary hypertension, 2.5 mg of bendroflumethiazide produces a maximal effect with minimum electrolyte disturbance. Higher doses cause other changes without additional antihypertensive qualities.

Side-effects/cautions

The thiazides may cause hypokalaemia and may aggravate diabetes and gout. They are contraindicated when there is hypokalaemia, natraemia or hypercalcaemia. Side-effects are postural hypertension, gastrointestinal effects, electrolyte disturbances and impotence. They act within a couple of hours of administration and last for up to 24 hours, so do not give them at bedtime.

Dosage   For oedema 5–10 mg in the morning or on alternate days, maintenance dose 1–3 times weekly, hypertension 2.5 mg per day.

Loop diuretics (furosemide and bumetanide)

They work by limiting reabsorption in the ascending limb of the loop of Henlé.

Indications

They are used in the treatment of pulmonary oedema due to ventricular failure, with intravenous administration giving relief of breathlessness, and can also be used for chronic heart failure. They can be used to treat hypertension if this is resistant to thiazides. There is no indication for routine potassium supplements when taking a thiazide or loop diuretic.

Side-effects/cautions

Hypokalaemia may develop as may hypotension. In renal failure, side-effects are hyponatraemia, hypocalcaemia and hypomagnesia.

Dosage Furosemide (Lasix®) 40 mg in the morning followed by maintenance dose of 20–40 mg, up to 80 mg in resistant conditions; bumetanide (Burinex®) 1 mg in the morning repeated after 8 hours, increase to maximum dose of 5 mg daily, 0.5 mg may suffice in older people.

Potassium-sparing diuretics (spironolactone, amiloride, triamterene)

These potentiate thiazide loop diuretics by antagonising aldosterone. Low doses may be helpful in severe heart failure and in primary hyperaldosteronism (Conn's syndrome).

Indications

The main indications are oedema and ascites (associated with cirrhosis of the liver, nephritic syndrome and malignant ascites).

Dosage 100–200 mg per day increasing to 400 mg a day if required (spironolactone is a specific aldosterone antagonist, amiloride and triamterene are other potassium-sparing diuretics); the trade name of spironolactone is Aldactone®; a useful combination is of a thiazide or loop diuretic with a potassium-sparing diuretic, although when indicated the drugs should be prescribed separately; if compliance is a big problem, combination preparations are available.

Calcium channel blockers

These drugs (amlodipine, diltiazem, felodipine, isradipine, lacidipine, lercanidipine, nicardipine, nifedipine, nimodipine and nisoldipine) interfere with the inward transfer of calcium through the cell membrane, influencing myocardial cells, with a consequent reduction in myocardial contractility.

Indications

They are used in the treatment of angina, hypertension and arrhythmia. There are significant differences between verapamil, diltiazem and the dihydropyridine calcium channel blockers. Verapamil and diltiazem should be avoided in heart failure as they further depress cardiac function. Calcium channel blockers do not reduce the risk of myocardial infarction in people with unstable angina, and drugs should be withdrawn gradually.

Verapamil is used for the treatment of angina, hypertension and arrhythmias. It reduces cardiac output and slows the heart rate, and may precipitate heart failure and exacerbate conduction disorders, and may cause hypotension. It should not be used in combination with beta-blockers.

Diltiazem is effective in angina, and the longer-acting formulation can be used for hypertension and may be used for patients where beta-blockers are contraindicated.

Nicardipine, amlodipine and felodipine depress cardiac activity much less than verapamil, and have no antiarrhythmic effect. All can be used in the treatment of angina associated with coronary vasospasm.

Isradipine, lacidipine, lercanidipine and nisoldipine have similar effects, with the first three indicated solely for the treatment of hypertension and the last two for additional symptoms of angina.

Nimodipine is confined to the use of prevention of vascular spasm following aneurysmal subarachnoid haemorrhage.

Side-effects/cautions

The most common side-effect of verapamil is constipation and those of the dihydropyridine antagonists are the side-effects associated with vasodilatation such as flushing, headache (tends to subside after a few days) and ankle swelling (only partially responsive to thiazides).

Dosage   Amlodipine (Istin®) 5 mg once daily, maximum dose 10 mg a day;

Diltiazem 60 mg twice a day increasing to maximum of 360 mg a day (longer-acting formulations available);

Felodipine 2.5 mg a day, maintenance 5–10 mg a day;

Isradipine 1.25 mg twice a day increased after 3–4 weeks to 5 mg twice a day, maintenance dose 2.5 or 5 mg a day;

Lacidipine 2 mg in the morning increased after 3–4 weeks to 4 mg and only rarely necessarily up to 6 mg;

Lercanidipine 10 mg daily increased after 3–4 weeks to 10 mg twice a day;

Nicardipine 20 mg three times a day increased after at least 3 days to 90 mg a day (usual range 60–120 mg a day);

Nifedipine (also known as Adalat®) doses vary according to the exact preparation, for non-proprietary nifedipine conditionally 5 mg three times a day, maximum 20 mg three times a day;

Nimodipine (specialist prescription);

Nisoldipine 10 mg a day before breakfast increasing no more than weekly to maximum of 40 mg;

Verapamil for arrhythmias 40–120 mg three times a day, for angina 80–120 mg three times a day, for hypertension 240–400 mg daily in up to three divided doses.

Beta-blockers

These are used for the treatment of hyperfusion and reduction of recurrence of myocardial infarction.

β-Adrenergic receptor-blocking drugs block the β-adrenergic receptors in the heart, peripheral vasculature, bronchi, pancreas and liver. Many are now available and are equally effective, but subtle differences between them will lead to a preference in one condition or another.

Indications

Intrinsic sympathomimetic activity represents the capacity of a beta-blocker to stimulate as well as to block adrenergic receptors. Examples of drugs with this action are oxprenolol, pindolol, acebutolol and celiprolol, which as a result cause less bradycardia and less coldness of the extremities. Some beta-blockers are water soluble (atenolol, celiprolol, nadolol and sotalol), and are less likely to enter the brain and therefore cause less sleep disturbance and nightmares, and as they are excreted by the kidneys, tend to accumulate where there is renal impairment. Beta-blockers with a relatively short duration of action have to be given 2–3 times a day, but some of these are available in modified-release formulations.

Side-effects/caution

Beta-blockers can slow the heart and depress the myocardium; hence, they are contraindicated in patients with second- or third-degree heart-block. Beta-blockers can precipitate asthma and should be avoided in patients with a history of bronchospasm.

Labetalol, celiprolol, carvedilol and nebivolol have an effect of lowering peripheral resistance, but there is nothing to suggest that they have advantages in treating hypertension.

Atenolol, isopropyl, metoprolol, nebivolol and acebutolol have less effect on bronchioreceptors and can be regarded as less cardioselective, but are certainly not cardiospecific. Their main actions are in reducing blood pressure, in relieving symptoms of angina (by reducing cardiac work) and in reducing the recurrence rate of myocardial infarction.

Angiotensin-converting enzyme inhibitors

Angiotensin-converting enzyme inhibitors (ACEIs) inhibit the conversion of angiotensin I to angiotensin II (captopril, cilazapril, enalapril maleate, fosinopril, imidapril, lisinopril, moexipril hydrochloride, perindopril, quinapril, ramipril and trandolapril).

Indications

They have a variety of indications including heart failure and hypertension, and, in more specialist centres, diabetic nephropathy. They may also have a place in the prophylaxis of cardiovascular events. They have a valuable role in all grades of heart failure, usually combined with a diuretic. ACEIs should be considered for hypertension when thiazides and/or beta-blockers are contraindicated, not tolerated or fail to control blood pressure.

Side-effects/cautions

ACEIs can cause very rapid falls of blood pressure, particularly in patients taking diuretics, when the first dose should preferably be at bedtime. ACEIs should only be initiated under specialist supervision, and are contraindicated in people with renal-vascular disease, and renal function should be monitored before and at a time after starting treatment. The main side-effects are hypotension, renal impairment and a persistent dry cough, as well as episodes of angio-oedema, rash and upper respiratory symptoms.

Dosage   Captopril 6.25 mg twice a day (first dose at bedtime) usually up to 25 mg, twice a day in hyptertension and up to 150 mg a day, under close medical supervision, for heart failure (other formulations include cilazapril, enalapril maleate, fosinopril, imidapril, lisinopril, moexipril hydrochloride, perindopril, quinapril, ramipril and trandolapril).

Angiotensin II receptor antagonists

Angiotensin II receptor antagonists (candesartan, irbesartan, losartan, eprosartan, olmesartan, telmisartan) add some more properties to the ACEIs but seem to be free of the persistent dry cough often associated with those. Roughly speaking, the cautions and contraindications are similar to those of the ACEIs with the side-effects usually being mild.

Dosage Older agents include candesartan (8–16 mg per day), irbesartan (75 mg per day, up to 300 mg), losartan (25 mg per day, up to 100 mg per day) and valsartan (40 mg a day, increasing after 4 weeks to 60 mg a day), with eprosartan, olmesartan (10 mg per day, up to 20 mg a day) and telmisartan (40 mg a day, increased after a month to 80 mg a day) being introduced more recently.

α-Adrenergic antagonists

These (prazosin, doxazosin, indoramin, terazosin) are used in the treatment of hypertension, and have postsynaptic alpha-blocking and vasodilating properties. They are also indicated for benign prostatic hyperplasia (urinary incontinence is a contraindication).

Dosage Preparations available are: prazosin (0.5 mg 2–3 times a day, last dose on retiring to bed, dose doubled after 3–7 days), doxazosin (1 mg a day increased after 1–2 weeks to 2 mg a day and after a similar time to 4 mg a day), indoramin (25 mg twice a day, increased by 25–50 mg every 2 weeks, maximum dose 200 mg) and terazosin (1 mg at bedtime with the dose doubled after 7 days, maximum 10 mg a day).

Nitrates

These have a useful role in angina, and although they are potent coronary vasodilators their principle benefit is as a result of a reduction in left ventricular work. Sublingual glyccrol trinitrate (GTN) is the most effective drug for providing rapid symptomatic relief of angina, with the effect lasting only up to 30 minutes. The aerosol spray is an alternative for rapid relief of symptoms for those in whom the sublingual preparation and the duration of action may be prolonged by modified-release and transdermal preparations. Isosorbide dinitrate is active sublingually and has a slower onset of action and may persist for several hours, up to 12 hours for the modified-release preparations. Isosorbide mononitrate, one of its metabolites, is licensed for angina prophylaxis, and modified-release formations are available. Many patients on the long-acting transdermal nitrates develop tolerance, with reduced therapeutic effects. Discontinuing some doses may prove to be of benefit.

Side-effects/cautions

Side-effects include flushing, headache and postural hypertension, which may limit the therapy.

They are contraindicted in severe hepatic renal impairment, hypothyroidism, head trauma and recent MI.

Dosage Thirty-seven different preparations of the three main agents are available as short-acting sprays or tablets, longer-acting tablets, transdermal patches and parenteral preparations. Non-proprietary GTN tablets prescribed in doses of 300 µg (should be discarded 8 weeks after opening) and an intravenous non-proprietary preparation are available, and longer-acting tablets and transdermal preparations are also available.

Isosorbide dinitrate should be given in doses of between 30 and 120 mg a day, and isosorbide mononitrate in doses orally starting at 10 mg twice a day for those who are nitrate naïve, with a maximum dose of 125 mg in divided doses.

Nicorandil

This is a potassium channel activator with a nitrate component, which has both arterial and vasodilating properties, and is licensed for the prevention and long-term treatment of angina.

Side-effects/cautions

Side-effects include cardiogenic shock, hypotension, headache and cutaneous vasodilatation, flushing, nausea, vomiting, dizziness and weakness.

Dosage 10 mg twice a day (half the dose if susceptible to headache), usual dose between 10–20 mg twice a day.

Digoxin

This is a cardiac glycoside which increases the force of myocardial contraction and reduces conductivity within the atrioventricular node. They are mostly used in the treatment of supraventricular tachycardias, especially to control ventricular response in atrial fibrillation. The ventricular rate should not be allowed to fall beneath 60, and digoxin is now rarely used for rapid control of heart rate (even with intravenous administration, response may take some hours). It can also be used in mild heart failure. Digoxin has a long half-life, and maintenance doses only need to be given once a day. Renal function determines the excretion of digoxin.

Side-effects/cautions

Recent myocardial infarction, sick sinus syndrome and thyroid disease are cautions, with many degrees of heart block and some supraventricular arrythmias being contraindications.

Dosage Between 1 and 1.5 mg can be given in divided doses over 24 hours, with maintenance between 62.5 and 500 µg a day, depending on heart rate response. Antibody treatments for the reverse of life-threatening overdose are available.

Phosphodiesterase inhibitors

Enoximone and milrinone are diphosphodiesterase inhibitors, exerting their effect on the myocardium; they may help with congestive heart failure and are given intravenously.

Amiodarone

Indications

This is used for the treatment of supraventricular and ventricular arrhythmias when other drugs are ineffective or contraindicated.

Side-effects/cautions

Sinus brachycardia and heart block are side-effects. It should only be initiated under specialist hospital provision. It has a very long half-life and only needs to be given once a day. Liver function and thyroid function tests should be carried out before treatment and every 6 months.

Dosage 200 mg three times a day for a week, reducing to 200 mg twice a day for a further week, with the maintenance dose being 200 mg a day.

Statins

The statins (atorvastatin, fluvastatin, pravastatin, rosuvastatin and simvastatin) inhibit one of the enzymes involved in cholesterol synthesis in the liver and are the most effective class of drugs in reducing low-density lipoproteins (LDLs) and cholesterol. There is good evidence that taking statins reduces myocardial infarction, cardiovascular episodes and mortality. They are now very widely used for the primary and secondary prevention of all cerebrovascular and cardiovascular events.

Their main use is obviously in the reduction of cholesterol, but while the risk of coronary events is not particularly accurately predicted from the level of cholesterol alone, it is still a reasonable target.

Side-effects/cautions

Liver disease or high alcohol intake should prompt the statins to be used with caution. Liver function tests should be done before and within 3 months of starting treatment and repeated every 6 months. Treatment should be discontinued if serum transaminase concentration is three times normal. Reversible myositis is a significant (but rare) side-effect of the statins, and treatment should be discontinued if creatine kinase is more than five times normal. Myalgia, myositis and myopathy have all been reported, and rhabdomyolysis associated with acute renal failure has been reported.

Dosage The level of cholesterol which should trigger prescription of a statin is said to be when the total concentration is 5 mmol/l or greater, and there is a coronary heart risk of 30% or greater over 10 years. The prescription of medication should be accompanied by advice and measures to improve life-style (e.g. losing weight, exercise, stopping smoking). The target cholesterol should be less than 5 mmol or a 25% reduction, whichever is lower, and for LDL cholesterol the target should be below 3 mmol or a 30% reduction, whichever is lower.

Preparations are atorvastatin (10 mg once a day), fluvastatin (20–40 mg a day in the evening; up to 80 mg a day may be required), pravastatin sodium (10 mg at night, increasing to 40 mg gradually by 10 mg every 4 weeks), rosuvastatin (10 mg a day, up to 20 mg a day after 4 weeks), and simvastatin (10 mg a day at night, increased by 10 mg every 4 weeks to a maximum of 80 mg).

ANALGESICS

Simple analgesics

Aspirin and paracetamol

Aspirin is the most commonly used non-opioid analgesic indicated for headache, transient musculoskeletal pain, dysmenorrhoea and pyrexia (in inflammatory conditions, a non-steroidal anti-inflammatory drug is usually preferred). Paracetamol is similar in efficacy to aspirin, but does not have any anti-inflammatory activity. It is less irritant to the stomach and is now generally preferred to aspirin. Overdose with paracetamol is particularly dangerous.

Side-effects/cautions

Paracetamol should be used with caution in hepatic and renal impairment. Side-effects are rare.

Dosage For an adult, paracetamol 0.5–1 g every 4–6 hours to a maximum of 4 g a day is the dosage of choice.

For aspirin 300–900 mg a day every 4–6 hours with a maximum of 4 g a day is indicated. Paracetamol and aspirin are part of a whole host of preparations on sale to the general public.

Nefopam hydrochloride (Acupan®)

Dosage For persistent pain, unresponsive to paracetamol or aspirin, 60 mg (elderly 30 mg) 3 times a day: usual range 30–90 mg a day.

Opioid analgesics

Opioid analgesics (morphine, diamorphine (heroin), codeine, buprenorphine, dipipanone, dextropropoxyphene, dihydrocodeine) are used to relieve moderate to severe pain, but repeated administration may cause dependence and tolerance.

Formulations

Morphine is the most valuable opioid analgesic for severe pain, although it frequently causes nausea and vomiting. It is the opiate of choice for the oral treatment of pain in palliative care, and can be given regularly every 4 hours or every 12–24 hours in a modified-release preparation. 10 mg every 4 hours by subcutaneous or muscular injection is the dose of choice, and oral solutions are available usually with 5 or 20 mg of morphine, with modified-release preparations containing between 5 and 30 mg.

Several other preparations are available:

Diamorphine (heroin) causes less nausea and hypotension than morphine, and its greater solubility allows smaller volumes to be injected; in palliative care, 5–10 mg every 4 hours is an appropriate dose;

Codeine is effective in the relief of mild to moderate pain, but constipation is a side-effect and makes long-term use inappropriate (30–60 mg every 4 hours, maximum 240 mg a day);

Buprenorphine has more opioid agonist properties; it has a longer duration of action than morphine and sublingually is an effective analgesic;.up to 8 hours is only partially reversed by naloxone (the standard treatment to reverse the central depressed effects of other opioids); 200–400 µg every 8 hours sublingually increasing to every 6 hours may be appropriate;

Dipipanone is less sedating than morphine, and is the only agent that contains an anti-emetic;

Dextropropoxyphene in combination with paracetamol (co-proxamol) has little advantage over paracetamol alone, and may be dangerous in overdose;

Dihydrocodeine has an effect similar to that of codeine (dose 30–60 mg every 4 hours).

Other agents include methadone, which is less sedating than morphine. Pethidine causes less constipation than morphine but is a less potent analgesic and is used particularly in labour pain; tramadol has an opioid effect and enhances serotonergic and adrenergic pathways, and is associated with fewer of the typical opioid side-effects (less respiratory depression, less constipation, less addiction, but confusional states may occur).

Side-effects/cautions

The most common side-effects are nausea, vomiting, constipation and drowsiness, with respiratory depression in larger doses. Drug interactions are particularly important with pethidine and the monoamine oxidase inhibitors.

Non-steroidal anti-inflammatory agents

In single doses, NSAIDs (ibuprofen, fenoprofen, flurbiprofen, ketoprofen, dexketoprofen, indometacin, naproxen) have analgesic activity comparable to paracetamol, and in regular full doses they have a lasting analgesic and anti-inflammatory effect, which makes them useful for the treatment of continuous pain. For example, paracetamol gives adequate pain control in osteoarthritis, but NSAIDs are more appropriate where there is inflammation of advanced osteoarthritis, back pain or soft tissue injury. The differences in anti-inflammatory activity between the various NSAIDs are small, and individual responses may determine which particular drug is used. The side-effects will determine the choice of drug.

The National Institute of Clinical Excellence (NICE) guidance on their use says that they should not be used as a routine and only preferred where there is a high risk of developing serious gastrointestinal disturbances (e.g. in those over the age of 65) and there is no justification for giving gastro-protective drugs to reduce gastrointestinal side-effects further.

Some 50 different preparations exist for various non-steroidal anti-inflammatory agents; recently, Vioxx was withdrawn because of an increased risk of cardiovascular events.

Side-effects/cautions

Ibuprofen is a propionic acid derivative, and has fewer side-effects than the other NSAIDs but weaker anti-inflammatory properties. Other propionic acid derivatives include naproxen; it has a low rate of side-effects. Fenbufen has a low risk of gastrointestinal bleeding but a higher risk of rashes. Fenoprofen, flurbiprofen, ketoprofen and dexketoprofen offer little to choose between them, and tiaprofenic acid has recently been associated with severe cystitis. Etoricoxib and valdecoxib are also available. According to Committee on Safety of Medicines (CSM) advice, azapropazone is associated with the highest risk of gastrointestinal side-effects, with ibuprofen the lowest and piroxicam, ketoprofen, indometacin, naproxen and diclofenac being associated with intermediate risks. The cyclo-oxygenase-2 drugs are associated with a lower risk.

Drugs with similar properties to those of propionic acid derivatives include azapropazone (more severe gastrointestinal toxicity and more likely to cause rashes – avoid sunlight because of photosensitivity reactions – 300 mg twice a day); diclofenac and aceclofenac are similar to naproxen; diflunisal has features in common with aspirin and has a long duration of action, allowing twice-daily administration. Indometacin is similar to naproxen but is associated with a high incidence of dizziness, headaches and gastrointestinal effects. Mefenamic acid has been associated with diarrhoea and blood disorders, nabumetone is comparable to naproxen, and piroxicam, sulindac, tenoxicam and tolfenamic acid all have minor pros and cons. Selective inhibitors of cyclo-oxygenase-2 including celecoxib, etodolac, meloxicam and rofecoxib are as effective as the NSAIDs and share the same range of side-effects, but there is an indication that there is a lower risk of gastrointestinal side-effects.

Dosage   Ibuprofen (1.2–1.8 g a day in 3–4 divided doses, preferably after food; modified-release preparations with codeine are available);

Fenbufen (300–600 mg, 3–4 times a day);

Naproxen (0.5–1 g daily in 1–2 divided doses);

Azapropazone (300 mg twice a day).

RESPIRATORY DRUGS

β_2-Agonists

Indications

Mild to moderate symptoms of asthma respond rapidly to the inhalation of selective short-acting β_2-agonists such as salbutamol or terbutaline. Salmeterol and formoterol are longer-acting agonists administered by inhalation, but should not be used for the relief of an acute asthma attack although may be added to existing steroid therapy. The short-acting agonists (salbutamol, terbutaline) should not be prescribed on a regular basis for patients with mild to moderate asthma, but the longer-acting agents may be of benefit. Pressurised metered-dose inhalers are a convenient and effective way of delivering drugs for mild to moderate asthma, and respirator (or nebuliser) solutions of salbutamol and terbutaline are used in the treatment of acute asthma. Intravenous preparations are available.

Side-effects/cautions

The agents should be used with caution in hypothyroidism and cardiovascular changes, and hypocalaemia is a side-effect, as are tremor, headache and palpitations.

Doses Salbutamol is given in a dose of 100–200 µg (1–2 puffs up to four times a day, and 2 mg 3–4 times a day by tablet). Terbutaline is given by aerosol with 1–2 puffs (250–500 µg, 3–4 times a day), with an initial dose of 2.5 mg, three times a day in tablet form.

Antimuscarinic bronchodilators

Ipratropium can provide short-term relief in chronic asthma, and can be used as an adjunct in nebulisation in life-threatening situations and may be effective in chronic obstructive pulmonary disease (20–40 mg 3–4 times a day by aerosol inhalation). Tiotropium is a longer-acting antimuscarinic bronchodilator used for maintenance treatment, and is not suitable for acute bronchospasm (inhalation, 80 µg of powder a day). Theophylline is a bronchodilator used for asthma and stable chronic obstructive pulmonary disease, and is metabolised in the liver. Plasma concentrations can vary in smokers and those with hepatic or heart failure. Theophylline is given by injection as aminophylline (a mixture of theophylline with ethylenediamine). It must be given very slowly, with blood levels taken, and tablets are available for maintenance treatment.

A wide variety of compound bronchodilator preparations and nebulisers are available.

Inhaled steroids

Corticosteroids are very effective in asthma and can reduce airway inflammation, but do not improve lung function. An inhaled steroid should be prescribed with a peak flow worse than 50% of the predicted value, or if the patient has had two or more exacerbations in a year, and it may useful as a therapeutic trial to separate those with asthma from those with a chronic obstructive disease. It must be used regularly for maximum benefit, and symptomatic response usually only occurs between 3 and 7 days after starting. The three main agents available – beclometasone diproprionate, budesonide and fluticasone – appear to be equally effective. Steroids should be used cautiously when there is a suggestion of tuberculosis, and parenteral administration may be needed at periods of stress, with paradoxical bronchospasm occasionally occurring.

Side-effects/cautions

Side-effects may include adrenal suppression (people on high doses should be given a steroid card). Doses of beclometasone range from $100\,\mu g$ 3–4 times a day to $800\,\mu g$ a day.

Cromoglycate

Sodium cromoglycate and nedocromil have a mode of action not completely understood, but may of benefit in allergic asthma. They are used as prophylactic agents, and are not effective in the treatment of an acute attack but may help in the prevention of exercise-induced asthma.

Dosage Aerosol inhalation is 10 mg, two puffs four times a day, which can be increased to eight times a day, and the dose of nedocromil is two puffs (4 mg, four times a day).

Leukotriene receptor antagonists

Montelukast and zafirlukast block the effects of cysteinyl leukotrienes in the airways, and may be effective in exercise-induced asthma. Doses of the former are 10 mg a day in the evening and of the latter 20 mg twice a day.

DISORDERS OF THE URINARY TRACT

Urinary retention

Chronic urinary retention is painless and usually long-standing, and selective α-adrenergic antagonists (alfuzosin, doxazosin, indoramin, prazosin, tamsulosin, terazosin) can relax smooth muscle in benign prostatic hyperplasia, producing an improvement in urinary outflow.

Side-effects/cautions

They may reduce blood pressure in people being prescribed antihypertensive agents who need particular supervision, and they are contraindicated in people with postural hypotension or micturation syncopy. Side-effects include drowsiness, hypotension, syncope and gastrointestinal disturbances, with hypersensitivity reaction also being reported. Parasympathomimetic agents (bethanechol and distigmine) promote detrusor muscle contraction but may have a very limited role in the relief of urinary retention.

Dosage   Preparations include alfuzosin (2.5 mg twice a day, up to 10 mg a day), doxazosin (1 mg a day, maintenance 2–4 mg a day), indoramin (20 mg at night in older people may be enough), prazosin (500 mg twice a day, up to 2 mg a day: NB first dose may cause collapse), tamsulosin (400 μg a day) and terazosin (1 mg at bedtime, doubled every 2 weeks to between 5 and 10 mg, NB first dose effect).

Urinary incontinence

This usually arises from detrusor instability, and a combination of drug treatment with non-drug approaches such as pelvic floor exercises and bladder draining is the treatment of choice. Antimuscarinic drugs (oxybutynin, tolterodine, flavoxate, propiverine, trospium) increase the capacity of the bladder and reduce contractions.

Side-effects/cautions

They should be avoided in people with myasthenia gravis, glaucoma, significant bladder outflow obstruction or urinary retention, ulcerative colitis or gastrointestinal problems such as obstruction or intestinal atony.

Dosage   These include oxybutynin (2.5–3 mg twice a day increased to 5 mg twice a day) which has a direct relaxant effect with side-effects (including dry mouth, constipation, blurred vision, drowsiness, nausea, vomiting, abdominal discomfort, palpitations, skin reactions and retention) that limit its use.

The modified-release version has fewer side-effects, similar to those of tolterodine (2 mg twice a day, reducing to 1 mg twice a day to minimise side-effects); flavoxate has fewer side-effects but is less effective (200 mg, three times a day), and propiverine (15 mg 1–3 times a day) and trospium (20 mg twice a day before food) are newer antimuscarinic agents.

NUTRITION AND BLOOD

Preparations should be given by mouth unless there are good reasons otherwise. Ferrous salts (ferrous fumarate, ferrous gluconate, ferrous succinate) are essentially all the same, but ferric salts are less well absorbed. Cost and side-effects determine choice.

Iron supplements

The oral dose of elemental iron for deficiency should be between 100 and 200 mg a day; ferrous sulphate 200 mg three times a day (up to 65 mg of elemental iron) may be effective for the treatment of mild iron-deficiency anaemia or for prophylaxis. Formulations include ferrous fumarate, ferrous gluconate and ferrous succinate, each of which have slightly different elemental iron contents. Modified-release preparations limit the amount of iron in the gastrointestinal tract at any one time, and can be used once a day. Side-effects are mostly gastrointestinal irritation, nausea and epigastric pain, and they can sometimes be the cause of constipation.

Vitamin supplements

Supplements of individual vitamins are generally available, and should be prescribed in the appropriate dosages. The British National Formulary lists vitamin A, vitamin B_2 (riboflavin), vitamin B_1 (thiamine), vitamin B_6 (piridoxine), nicotinamide, vitamin C, vitamin D, vitamin A and vitamin K. These are generally not used as dietary supplements, but may be prescribed to prevent or treat deficiency. Their use as a tonic is of unproven value, and megavitamin therapy with vitamin C or some of the vitamin B complex is unscientific and could be harmful. Multivitamin preparations such as vitamin capsules are available, and also exist in droplet form.

Nutritional supplements

These consist of items available that appear in the British National Formulary under Appendix 7 (borderline substances – they can be prescribed as long as they are regarded by a doctor as safe, the patient can be monitored, supervision is available and they are for the management of a specified condition). Our favourite is 'rectified spirit'. Where the therapeutic qualities of alcohol are required, 'rectified spirit' (suitably flavoured and diluted) should be prescribed. Agents in this category include Maxijul®, available for malnutrition and malabsorption, which contains carbohydrate and a number of sugars.

DIABETES

Diabetes mellitus occurs because of a lack of insulin or a resistance to its action. It is divided into type 1 diabetes, also known as insulin-dependent diabetes mellitus, which is due to an insufficiency of insulin following autoimmune destruction of the pancreatic beta cells, and type 2 diabetes, non-insulin dependent diabetes, due to reduced secretion of insulin or to peripheral resistance to its action. Although patients may be controlled by diet alone, many require oral antidiabetic drugs and/or insulin to maintain satisfactory control. The prescription and understanding of insulin is a specialist field, being divided into short-acting insulins such as soluble insulin and intermediate- and long acting insulins.

Oral antidiabetic drugs

These are used for the treatment of type 2 diabetes mellitus, and should only be prescribed if the patient fails to respond adequately to 3 months' restriction of energy and carbohydrate intake with an increase in physical activity.

Sulphonylureas

These act by augmenting insulin secretion, and therefore are only effective when there is some residual activity. They may cause hypoglycaemia and are considered for patients who are not overweight or in whom metformin (see below) is not appropriate. The long-acting suphonylureas, chlorpropamide and glibenclamide, are associated with a greater risk of hypoglycaemia, and should probably therefore be avoided in older people.

The shorter-acting alternatives, gliclazide (40–80 mg a day adjusted up to 100 mg, maximum 320 mg a day) and tolbutamide (0.5–1.5 g, maximum 2 g daily in divided doses with or immediately after breakfast) should be preferred. Chlorpropamide seems to have more side-effects and is no longer recommended.

Side-effects/cautions

Sulphonylureas can encourage weight gain. Caution is needed in the elderly and in those with mild to moderate hepatic and renal impairment because of the hazard of hypoglycaemia, and should be avoided in severe hepatic and renal impairment. Side-effects include gastrointestinal and those of hypoglycaemia. (Chlorpropamide is famously associated with facial flushing after drinking.)

Metformin

This is the only available biguanide, which has a different mode of action from the sulphonylureas and exerts its effect by decreasing gluconeogenesis and increasing peripheral utilisation of glucose – it acts only in the presence of endogenous insulin. It is the drug of first choice in overweight patients if strict dieting has failed. Hypoglycaemia usually does not occur, but gastrointestinal side-effects can be a problem.

Dosage 500 mg with breakfast for 1 week, then with breakfast and the evening meal for 1 week, and then with breakfast, lunch and the evening meal up to a maximum of 2–3 g per day.

Other antidiabetic agents include acarbose, an inhibitor of intestinal α-glucosidases, which delays the digestion and absorption of starch; nateglinide and repaglinide, which stimulate insulin release; and pioglitazone and rosiglitazone, which reduce peripheral insulin resistance.

HYPOTHYROIDISM

Thyroid hormones

Levothyroxine sodium (thyroxin sodium) is the treatment of choice for maintenance therapy. The initial dose should not exceed 100 μg a day, preferably before breakfast, or 25–50 μg in older patients with cardiac disease, increased at intervals of a month by 25–50 μg, with a maintenance dose of between 100 and 200 μg.

Liothyronine sodium has a similar action, but is more rapidly metabolised and has a rapid effect. It can be used in severe hypothyroid states and is available intravenously. Prescription of drugs for thyrotoxicosis is a specialist field.

PARKINSON'S DISEASE

Drugs for Parkinson's disease should be initiated under the supervision of a physician specialising in the disorder. Treatment is not usually started until symptoms are of sufficient severity to interfere with activities of daily living.

Dopamine agonists

The dopamine receptor agonists bromocriptine (1.25 mg at night in week 1, doubled in week 2, 2.5 mg twice a day in week 3, three times a day in week 4 and then increasing by 2.5 mg every 1–2 weeks according to response to a range of between 10 and 40 mg a day, taken with food), cabergoline, lisuride, pergolide, pramipexole and ropinirole have a direct action on dopamine receptors and are usually started first, but can be used with L-dopa in more advanced disease. Apomorphine is a potent dopamine agonist which may be of help in advanced disease, but is only prescribed under specialist supervision and with cover with an antiemetic.

Side-effects/cautions

They cause fewer motor complications but more neuropsychiatric complications than L-dopa, but are probably slightly less effective. Fibrotic reactions (pulmonary, retroperitoneal, pericardial) have been described with the ergot-based receptor agonists (all the above except pramipexole and ropinirole) and ESR serum creatinine. Chest X-rays should be carried out before treatment and patients monitored for symptoms throughout. Excessive daytime sleepiness and sudden onset of sleep can occur with co-careldopa, co-beneldopa and the dopamine receptor agonists, and patients should be advised of this, with a warning not to drive or operate machinery (although hardly anyone in the UK operates machinery any more).

L-dopa

L-dopa is the amino acid precursor of dopamine, and boosts the level of the neurotransmitter in the striatum. It is given with an extracerebral dopa-decarboxylase inhibitor to reduce peripheral conversion of L-dopa to dopamine, and therefore limits the peripheral side-effects such as nausea and vomiting. Benserazide is the inhibitor in co-beneldopa (dose expressed in terms of L-dopa dose: initiate 50 mg once or twice a day, increasing by 50 mg every 3–4 days according to response; for example, Madopar® contains 50 mg of L-dopa, 12.5 mg of benserazide, and is also available in 125- and 250-mg formulations and may be dispersed in water or orange squash – not orange juice – or swallowed whole; modified-release version is available), and carbidopa in co-careldopa. The equivalent of co-careldopa is Sinemet®, which should be given in a similar regime and is available as 62.5, 110, 125 and 275 mg). A modified-release version is available. These preparations are useful in people who are elderly and frail with co-morbid illness and severe symptoms. Therapy should be initiated at a low dose and increased in small steps, and the final dose should be the minimum needed, and intervals between doses should be bespoke. Entacapone prevents the peripheral breakdown of L-dopa and may be helpful with co-careldopa and co-beneldopa, and there is end-of-dose deterioration.

Side-effects/cautions

L-dopa treatment has been associated with the development of motor complications such as fluctuations in response, and dyskinesias characterised by changes in on/off periods and in dose deterioration.

Selegiline (2.5 mg a day up to 10 mg a day) is a monoamine-oxidase-B inhibitor and can be used in conjuction with L-dopa to reduce end-of-dose deterioration. It can be used early and may delay the need for L-dopa, but other drugs are preferred. Other drugs should be avoided in combination with L-dopa when there is postural hypotension.

Amantadine (100 mg a day up to a maximum of 400 mg a day) has modest anti-parkinsonian effects. It improves bradykinesia as well as tremor and rigidity, but tolerance may occur and confusion and hallucinations have been reported.

Antimuscarinic drugs

These exert an anti-parkinsonian action by reducing the central cholinergic excess which occurs as result of dopamine deficiency. They are generally not useful in idiopathic Parkinson's disease, they may exacerbate cognitive impairment. They may be of use in countering the side-effects of neuroleptic drugs, but in practice are rarely used in the elderly because of their tendency to cause confusion.

Benzatropine, procyclidine and trihexyphenidyl (benzhexol) are examples of the drugs, and benzatropine and procyclidine can be given parenterally to counter the effect of acute drug dystonias. The dose of procyclidine is 2.5 mg, three times a day to a maximum of 30 mg a day, with an aspiration to find the lowest possible dose in elderly people. The benzatropine dose is 0.5–1 mg a day at bedtime, gradually increased to a maximum of 6 mg but usually in a range of 1–4 mg, again with the lower end of the dose range preferred for elderly people.

Side-effects/cautions

The drugs may cause confusional states.

EPILEPSY

Preventing the occurrence of seizure activity is the goal of antiepileptic treatment. The frequency of administration is determined by the half-life of the drugs, which are usually given twice a day. Combination therapy is only indicated after monotherapy with several drugs has failed, as toxicity and drug interactions are much greater.

Partial seizures with or without secondary generalisation

Carbamazepine, lamotrigine, sodium valproate and phenytoin can be used as monotherapy for tonic–clonic seizures and for partial (focal) seizures. An alternative is oxcarbazepine; phenobarbital (phenobarbitone) and primidone are effective but are more sedating.

Generalised seizures

Tonic–clonic (grand mal): drugs of choice are carbamazepine, lamotrigine, phenytoin and sodium valproate.

Absence seizures (petit mal): ethosuximide and sodium valproate are the drugs of choice and lamotrigine (unlicensed for this) may be of help.

Atypical absence, atonic and tonic seizures: these are usually seen in childhood and the treatment is best dealt with by specialists.

Carbamazepine and oxcarbazepine

Carbamazepine is the drug of choice for complex partial seizures and for tonic–clonic seizures secondary to a focal discharge. It has a wider therapeutic index than phenytoin and fewer side-effects. Carbamazepine should be initiated at a low dose and built up at increments of between 100 and 200 mg every 2 weeks.

Side-effects/cautions

Blood disorders are a particular problem, as are psychotic states and rashes.

Dosage   Initial dose is 500 mg a day increased by increments of 250 mg every 7 days to between 1 and 1.5 g, maximum 2 g.

Gabapentin

Precautions include a history of psychotic illness, and it should be used sparingly in the elderly. Sudden withdrawal should be avoided.

Dosage   300 mg on the first day increasing by 300 mg a day to a maximum of 2.4 g a day, usually 0.9–1.2 g.

Lamotrigine

Hepatic, renal and clotting parameters should be monitored and rash, fever, flu-like symptoms, drowsiness or worsening of seizures should prompt withdrawal. Anaemia, bruising or infection should be mentioned specifically to the patient to watch out for.

Dosage   25 mg a day for 14 days, increased to 50 mg for a further 14 days, to a maximum of 50–100 mg.

Phenobarbitone

This should be used with caution in the elderly. It may cause respiratory depression, and sudden withdrawal should be avoided.

Dosage   60–180 mg at night.

Phenytoin

As with phenobarbitone, the initial dose is 120 mg at bedtime increased by that dose every 3 days to 500 mg in two divided doses to a maximum of 1.5 g a day. It should be used with caution in hepatic impairment, avoiding sudden withdrawal, and blood counts are recommended.

Dosage   150–300 mg a day as a single dose or two divided doses up to a maximum of 500 mg a day.

Valproate

Liver function should be monitored before therapy and every 6 months after that, and any bleeding tendency should be assessed. Blood disorders and pancreatitis are side-effects, and the patient should be monitored for their presence. Gastric irritation, nausea and ataxia may occur.

Dosage   600 mg a day in two divided doses up to maximum of 2.5 g. Usual maintenance is between 1 and 2 g a day.

GASTROINTESTINAL SYSTEM

Confirming the presence of *Helicobacter pylori* is recommended before starting eradication treatment. Acid inhibition combined with antibacterial treatment is highly effective, and reinfection is rare. One week of triple therapy comprises a proton pump inhibitor, amoxicillin and either clarithromycin or metronidazole. This eradicates the infection in over 90% of cases, and there is usually no need to continue with a proton pump inhibitor or H_2 receptor antagonist unless haemorrhage or perforation complicates the ulcer. A 2-week triple therapy regime increases the chance of eradication, but poor compliance is linked to side-effects and 2-week dual therapy with a proton pump inhibitor and single antibacterial agent is recommended.

Most gastric ulcers and duodenal ulcers are caused either by nonsteroidal anti-inflammatory agents or by infection with *H. pylori*.

H_2 receptor antagonists

All H_2 receptor antagonists heal gastric and duodenal ulcers by reducing gastric acid via a lowering of histamine H_2 receptors. In addition to healing ulcers caused by infection, they can relieve gastro-oesophageal reflux and the Zollinger–Ellison syndrome and can promote healing in NSAID-associated ulcers.

Side-effects/cautions

The drugs should be used with caution in hepatic and renal impairment. Always check the drug history of an older person.

Side-effects include diarrhoea and other gastrointestinal disturbances, altered liver function tests, headache, dizziness, rash and tiredness.

Dosage Cimetidine is taken 400 mg twice a day with breakfast or 800 mg at night for 4 weeks, increasing to a maximum of 400 mg four times a day.

Ranitidine is given in a dose of 150 mg twice a day or 300 mg at night. Other H_2 antagonists are famotidine (40 mg at night for up to 8 weeks and 20 mg at night as a maintenance dose) and nizatidine (300 mg twice a day or 300 mg in the evening, with a maintenance dose of 150 mg in the evening).

All H_2 antagonists are available over the counter.

Proton pump inhibitors

Proton pump inhibitors are omeprazole (20 mg once a day), esomeprazole (20 mg twice a day), lansoprazole (30 mg twice a day), pantoprazole (40 mg twice a day) and rabeprazole (20 mg twice a day). They inhibit gastric acid by blocking the hydrogen–potassium adenosine triphosphatase enzyme system (the 'proton pump') of the gastric parietal cell. They are effective as a short-term treatment for gastric and duodenal ulcers and gastro-oesophageal reflux. They may also be used in the prevention and treatment of NSAID-associated ulceration.

Side-effects/cautions

The drugs should be used with caution in people with liver disease and may mask symptoms of gastric cancer. Side-effects include gastrointestinal disturbances (nausea, vomiting, abdominal pain, flatulence, diarrhoea, constipation), headache and dizziness.

Antacids and semethicone

Antacids usually contain aluminium or magnesium compounds, and may cause improvement in symptoms in dyspepsia and gastro-oesophageal reflux (in the absence of erosions), where symptoms are expected to arise between meals and at bedtime. Doses are 10 ml three or four times a day, and liquid preparations are more effective than solid. Magnesium-containing antacids tend to be more laxative, and aluminium-containing ones tend to be more constipating. Sodium bicarbonate should no longer be used for the relief of dyspepsia, or bismuth-containing antacids because of the absorption of bismuth, which can be neurotoxic. An antifoaming agent, simethicone, can be added to relieve flatulence.

Alginate-containing antacids form a raft that floats on the surface of the stomach contents to reduce reflux, and may be helpful in mild symptoms of gastro-oesophageal reflux disease (the best known is Gaviscon® which can be taken in a dose of 1–2 tablets chewed after meals and at bedtime). More than 35 indigestion preparations are available over the counter, many of which are household names.

Laxatives

Before prescribing laxatives, it is essential to ensure that the patient is constipated, and that any diarrhoea is an overflow phenomenon as a result of that. Laxatives can be divided into a number of different types.

Bulk-forming types relieve constipation by increasing the faecal mass, which stimulates peristalsis. They are of particular value in those with small hard stools, and fibre should be increased in the diet. As a first line of treatment there must be adequate fluid intake, and unprocessed wheat bran taken with food or fruit juice is a most effective bulk-forming preparation. Methylcellulose (3–6 tablets a day), ispaghula (Fybogel®, one sachet or two 5-ml spoonfuls a day) and sterculia (1–2 sachets twice a day) are useful when bran cannot be tolerated.

Stimulant laxatives include bisacodyl (5–10 mg at night), senna (2–4 tablets) and dantron (1–2 tablets at bedtime; risk of malignancy with dantron). Powerful stimulants such as cascara and castor oil are obsolete. Docusate sodium (500 mg a day in divided doses) has a dual action as a stimulant and a softening agent.

Some faecal softeners are still used, such as liquid paraffin (10–30 ml – should not be taken immediately before going to bed), and arachis oil enemas lubricate and soften impacted faeces.

Osmotic laxatives

These work by increasing the amount of water in the large bowel or by drawing fluid from the body, or retaining fluid already there.

Purgatives such as magnesium hydroxide (25–50 ml) are useful occasionally, but adequate fluid intake should be maintained. Magnesium salts are particularly helpful when rapid evacuation is required, and sodium salts should be avoided as they may give rise to sodium and water retention. Salts are available in enema form.

Antibiotics

The choice of drugs should be determined by characteristics of the patient (e.g. history of allergy, renal and hepatic function) and the known or likely organism involved. It is likely that local policies exist for the range of antibiotics which can be prescribed without resource to a specialist. This section concentrates on those infections seen most commonly in old age psychiatry.

Exacerbation of chronic chest disease

Amoxicillin (250 mg every 8 hours) or ampicillin (between 250 mg and 1 g every 6 hours, depending on the seriousness of the infection), or tetracyclin (250 mg every 6 hours, up to 500 mg every 6 hours in serious infections) or erythromycin (250–500 mg every 6 hours depending on severity), can be used.

Hospital-acquired pneumonia

A broad-spectrum cephalosporin such as cefotaxime or ceftazidime (parenteral use only), or an anti-pseudomonal penicillin such as ticarcillin or piperacillin (parenteral use only), can be prescribed.

Urinary tract infections

Trimethoprim (200 mg every 12 hours, watch for blood disorder), amoxicillin (see above), nitrofurantoin (50 mg every 6 hours with food), oral cephalosporin (treatment for 3 days usually adequate, but 7 days may be required) or cefalexin (200 mg every 6 hours or 500 mg every 8 hours) can be used.

Conjunctivitis

Use chloramphenicol or gentamicin eye drops (apply one drop every 2 hours then reduce frequency and continue for 48 hours after healing; for eye ointment, apply three or four times a day).

7   Further reading

British National Formulary. London: British Medical Association and Royal Pharmaceutical Society.
(This is an essential adjunct to clinical practice and provides easy access to key information. You cannot prescribe safely without this!)

Runge MS, Greganti MA, eds. Netter's Internal Medicine. Icon Learning Systems, 2003.
(This is not the most comprehensive textbook of internal medicine available but it is stunningly illustrated, extremely readable and reasonably priced.)

Jones HR, ed. Netter's Neurology. Icon Learning Systems, 2005.
(Like Netter's Internal Medicine, this book is richly illustrated, has an easy style and is reasonably priced.)

Ross RT. How to Examine the Nervous System. Appleton and Lange. 1999.
(This is an exceptionally clear and concise book with plenty of line drawings. It is easy to read and tells you what you need to do. It is very reasonably priced, too!)

8   Appendix

GENERAL NEUROLOGICAL EXAMINATION

Cranial nerves

I:	Smell
II:	Fundi
	Visual fields
	Acuity
III, IV, VI:	Pupils: swinging torch test
	Lid movement
	Eye movements
	Nystagmus
V:	Facial sensation
VII:	Facial symmetry and movement
VIII:	Hearing
IX, X:	Uvula and palate movements
	Gag reflex
XI:	Neck musculature
XII:	Tongue position, movement, strength

Motor/muscle

Posture
Tone
Movement
Atrophy
Fasciculation

Reflexes

Deep tendon reflexes and plantars
Superficial reflexes
Frontal release (primitive) reflexes

Sensory examination

Light touch
Pinprick
Position
Tremor
Other abnormal movements

Neck

Movements
Pain/tenderness
Head rolling/side-lying tests

Gait and posture

Standing
    eyes open
    eyes closed
    displacement
Walking
Arm swing
Turning
Base
Spasticity

Back

Spine shape
Straight leg raising

Index

abdomen,
  basic physical examination 13
  signs of disease in 15
abdominal pain, *see* pain
absence seizures 103, 240
acidosis in renal failure 52
acoustic neuroma 111
actinic keratoses 182
Addison's disease and hypercalcaemia 28
α-adrenergic antagonists for cardio-vascular disease 225
Adults with Incapacity (Scotland) Act 2000 22–4
advance directives 25
adverse reactions to drugs 217
aging processes and how they affect medicine 1
akinesia, examination for 19
akinetic mutism 74
albumin,
  and calcium abnormalities 28
  tests for 37
alkaline phosphatase 38
  and calcium abnormalities 28
altered mental state 60
amiodarone for cardiovascular disease 227
anaemia,
  definition 31
  haematological indices 32
  history taking for 31
  macrocytic 33
  medical examination for 32
  microcytic 33
  normocytic 33
  symptoms of 31
analgesics, *see* pain
angiotensin-converting enzyme inhibitors,
  for cardiovascular disease 224
  use in heart failure 125

angiotensin II receptor antagonists,
  for cardiovascular disease 224
  use in heart failure 125
angular cheilosis 14
ankles, basic physical examination 13
antacids 243
antibiotics 244
anticonvulsants, use in pain 156
antidepressants, use in pain 156
antimuscarinic bronchodilators, 232, 239
anus, bleeding from 190, 191
appearance, general 11
apraxic changes in gait 115
arms, signs of disease in 16
arousal, neuroanatomy of 61
arteritis,
  cranial 119
  giant cell 119
  temporal 119
artificial nutrition and hydration, withdrawal of 26
aspirin 228
  for cardiovascular disease 218
  use in hypertension 130
asteatotic dermatitis 182
asthma, nebuliser therapy for 60
ataxia 114
  examination for 19
atonic seizures 103
atypical presentation 2

back pain, *see* pain
balance,
  assessment of 18
  maintenance of 92
  physiology of 89
  somatosensory system 92
  vestibular system 89, 90
  visual system 90, 91
basal cell carcinoma 183

benign paroxysmal positional vertigo
108, 109
benign prostatic hypertrophy 55
examination for 55
symptoms 55
treatment 56
best interests 26
biliary obstruction 40
bilirubin,
causes of raised levels 37
tests for 37
biochemical profile for diagnosis 5
biochemical results for calcium abnormalities 27
blackouts 98, 99
causes of 99
cf sleep 99
premonitory symptoms 99
symptoms and diagnosis 99
bleeding, rectal 190, 191
blistering diseases 183
β₂-agonists for respiratory problems
232
β-blockers,
for cardiovascular disease 223
use in heart failure 125
blood lipids, for diagnosis 5
blood pressure,
basic physical examination 13
see also hypertension; hypotension
brain, internal herniations of 72
breathlessness,
acute 57
causes 57
evaluation of 57
nebuliser therapy 60
oxygen therapy 59
stridor 58
tension pneumothorax 59
treatment of 58
chronic severe hypoxaemia 59
bruits, signs of disease 15

calcitonin 48
calcium,
abnormal results for 27
hypercalcaemia 28
hypocalcaemia 29
role of 27
calcium channel blockers for cardiovascular disease 221
calf pain, see pain

caloric testing 71
cancer,
basal cell carcinoma 183
rectal in dementia patient 209
shadows on lung 209
squamous carcinoma 189
capacity,
in England/Wales/Northern Ireland
24
in Scotland 24
legal test of 24
Mental Capacity Bill 25
carbamazepine use in epilepsy 240
cardiovascular disease,
α-adrenergic antagonists for 225
amiodarone 227
angiotensin-converting enzyme
inhibitors for 224
angiotensin II receptor antagonists
for 224
aspirin for 218
β-blockers for 223
calcium channel blockers for 221
clopidogrel for 219
digoxin for 226
dipyridamole for 219
diuretics for 220
nicorandil for 226
nitrates for 225
phosphodiesterase inhibitors for
227
questions on for medical history 12
statins for 227
cellulitis 165, 183
central sleep apnoea 67
cerebellar tremor 199
chest disease, exacerbation of chronic
245
chest pain, see pain
cholesterol, see also lipids
chorea 115
Huntington's 199
clopidogrel for cardiovascular disease
219
Clostridium difficile 86, 87
cluster headaches 119
co-morbidity,
atypical presentation of disease and
2
prevalence in elderly 1
colon, bleeding from 190, 191
coma 60, 67, 67–75

akinetic mutism 74
central nervous system causes 74
cf sleep 63
diagnosis 73
examination of patient 69, 70
Glasgow Coma Scale 69
immediate measures in 68
internal herniations of brain 72
locked-in syndrome 75
management 73
medical history and 73
oculocephalic responses in 71
opisthotonos 72
posture in 72
compliance with drugs 218
conjunctivitis 245
consciousness,
akinetic mutism 74
blackouts 98, 99
caloric testing 71
coma 67–75
coma/sleep/altered mental state 60
definition and components of 61
diminished 67
drop attacks 100
examination of unconscious patient
69–71
fits/epilepsy 102–5
funny turns 106–12
Glasgow Coma Scale 69
internal herniations of brain 72
locked-in syndrome 75
management of head injury 122,
123
management of unconscious patient
68
medical history and coma diagnosis
73
neuroanatomy of arousal 61
oculocephalic responses 71
opisthotonos 72
posture and 72
questions concerning loss of 98
soporose cf stuporose patients
69
stratification of levels 68
vertebrobasilar ischaemia 100, 101
consent,
Adults with Incapacity (Scotland)
Act 2000 22–4
definition 21

in England/Wales/Northern Ireland
21, 22
in Scotland 22
problems with in dementia 20
refusal of treatment 211
constipation 75–7
drug causes of 76
laxatives 244
mechanisms of 75
symptoms of 75
treatments 76, 77
contact dermatitis 184
COPD, nebuliser therapy 60
core temperature 95
cough,
causes of 77
examination for 78
history of 78
investigations for 78
management 79
cramp 165
cranial arteritis 119
creatinine,
and calcium abnormalities 28
in acute renal failure 52
renal disease and 51
cromoglycate 233

Data Protection Act 22
deep vein thrombosis 166, 167
dehydration 79, 80, 211
dementia,
feeding problems in 194
neurological examination in 19
oxygen therapy compliance in 60
rectal cancer in 209
depression,
rheumatoid arthritis and 210
weight loss and tiredness in 205
dermatitis,
asteatotic 182
contact 184
seborrhoeic 188
diabetes mellitus 80–5
chronic renal failure in 53
description 80, 81
diabetic ketoacidosis 84
diagnosis 81
emergencies in 84, 85
hyperosmolar non-ketotic diabetic
coma 84
hypoglycaemia 84

long-term complications 81
management 81, 82
metformin for 237
monitoring 82, 83
nutrition in 84, 85
oral antidiabetic drugs 236
sulphonylureas for 236
symptoms 80
treatment choices 83
diabetic ketoacidosis 84
diagnosis,
    cf problem management 7
    golden rules of 4
diarrhoea 85–9
    acute,
        causes of 85, 86
        management of 87
    chronic,
        causes of 87, 88
        fatty 88
        inflammatory 88
        watery 87
    drugs as a cause of 88, 89
    underlying mechanisms of 86
digestion, questions on for medical
        history 12
digoxin,
    for cardiovascular disease 226
    use in heart failure 125
dipyridamole for cardiovascular dis-
        ease 219
diuretics,
    for cardiovascular disease 220
    use in heart failure 124
dizziness,
    differential diagnosis 108
    management 111, 112
do not resuscitate orders 26
dopamine agonists for Parkinsonism
        238
drop attacks 100
    causes of 100
    see also falls
drugs,
    action in elderly 1
    adverse reactions to 217
    antiemetics 146
    as cause of constipation 76
    as cause of diarrhoea 88, 89
    compliance 218
    fevers and 94, 95
    golden rules of prescribing 6

hepatocellular damage and 39
ototoxic 110, 111
pharmacodynamics 217
pharmacokinetics of 216
prescribing in elderly 215
questions on for medical history 12
risk vs. benefit 217
skin eruptions and 184
taking medications 196
duty of care 19
dysequilibrium 106
dystonia 114, 115, 199

entrapment neuropathy 173
eosinophilia 35, 36
epilepsy 102–5
    carbamazepine/oxcarbazepine for
        240
    drug treatments for 240
    gabapentin for 241
    lamotrigine for 241
    management of 104, 105
    phenobarbitone for 241
    phenytoin for 241
    valproate for 242
erythema multiforme 185
erythrocyte sedimentation rate,
    for diagnosis 5
    high 208
essential tremor 198
European Convention on Human
        Rights, articles involved in med-
        ical practice 21
euvolaemia 45, 46
examination, see also medical examina-
        tion; neurological examination
experience, importance of in physi-
        cians 3
exploding-head syndrome 120
extrapyramidal changes in gait 114
eyes, signs of disease in 15

face, basic physical examination 13
faecal incontinence 136, 137
faints 98
falls,
    approaches to 93, 94
    causes of 89–93
    conditions associated with 93
    incidence of 92
    management of patient after 93, 94
    physiology of balance 89

feeding,
amount and rate 196
dining environment 196
food consistency 196
position for 195
safety in 195
saliva management 196
taking medications 196
feet,
basic physical examination 13
common disorders in elderly 17
fever 94–7
causes of 95, 96
diagnosis of infection from top
down 95, 96
investigations used in diagnosis 96,
97
management 97
medical examination in 96
fingers, signs of disease in 16
fistula, perilymphatic 111
fits 97, 102
epilepsy and 102
see also consciousness; seizures
fixed drug eruptions 185
focal signs 19
folic acid for diagnosis 5
foot drop 114
full blood count,
for diagnosis 5
haematological indices and
anaemia 32
in leucocytosis 33, 34
funny turns 97, 106–111
assessment of 106, 107
differential diagnosis of dizziness
108
medical examination for 107
medical history 107

gabapentin use in epilepsy 241
gait 112–16
antalgic changes in 115
apraxic changes in 115
assessment of 18, 116
ataxia 114
causes of abnormal 112, 113
cautious 115
chorea and 115
extrapyramidal changes in 114
foot drop 114
hemiplegic changes 113, 114

myopathic changes 113
neuropathic changes 113
normal 112
Parkinsonism and 114
progressive supranuclear palsy and
115
psychogenic changes 116
spastic changes 113
subcortical changes in 115
gastro-oesophageal reflux disease
161
gastrointestinal ulcers 242
Gélineau syndrome 67
genitofemoral neuralgia 162
get-up-and-go test 18
giant cell arteritis 119
Glasgow Coma Scale 69
glomerulonephritis 53
γ-glutamyl transpeptidase 38
Grave's disease 50
gynaecological problems 116, 117
changes with age 116
postmenopausal bleeding 117
uterovaginal prolapse 117
vaginal discharge 117
vulval disorders 116, 117

H₂ receptor antagonists for gastrointestinal ulcers 242
haematological indices 32, 34
haemoglobin, abnormalities of 31
haemolysis 38
hand pain, see pain
hands,
basic physical examination 13
signs of disease in 16
Hashimoto's disease 49
Hashimoto's encephalopathy 51
head, basic physical examination 14
head injury 111, 121–3
headache 117–21
acute new-onset 118
cluster 119
exploding-head syndrome 120
hypnic 120
medication and 121
meningitis 118
post-herpetic neuralgia 121
raised intracranial pressure and
118
recurrent 119
subarachnoid haemorrhage 119

temporal/giant cell/cranial arteritis 119
temporomandibular neuralgia 121
tension-type 120
trigeminal neuralgia 120
hearing,
    basic physical examination 13
    signs of disease in 15
heart failure 123–7
    common problems in patients with 126
    investigations for 124
    management 124
    monitoring 125
    symptoms 123, 124
hepatocellular disease 39
hiccups 127
history, *see* medical history
hospital-acquired pneumonia 245
Human Rights Act 20
    major implications for health care 21
Huntington's chorea 199
hypercalcaemia,
    causes of 28
    symptoms of 28
hyperkalaemia 41
    causes of 41, 42
    in heart failure 126
    in renal failure 52
    management 42
hyperlipidaemia,
    causes of 30
    management 30
    primary prevention 30
hypernatraemia,
    causes of 45
    management 46
hyperosmolar non-ketotic diabetic coma (HONK) 84
hypersomnias 67
hypertension 128–32
    aetiology 128, 129
    complications of 130
    guidelines on treatment 129, 130
    in diabetes mellitus 82
    in elderly 128
    malignant/accelerated 132
    management of 129
    treatments,

ABCD rule of medication 131, 132
    life-style advice 131
    when to treat 129–31
hyperthyroidism,
    definition 50
    treatment 50
hypervitaminosis D and hypercalcaemia 28
hypervolaemia 45, 47
hypnic headache 120
hypocalcaemia,
    causes of 29
    symptoms of 29
hypoglycaemia 84, 85
hypokalaemia 43
    causes of 43
    management 43
hyponatraemia,
    causes of 46
    features of 47
    management of 48
hypotension 133–5
    definition 133
    in heart failure 126
    management 133, 134
    postural 134
        causes of 133
        treatments for 135
hypothyroidism 49
    definition of 49
    presentation 50
    treatment 49, 237
hypoventilation, nocturnal 67
hypovolaemia 45, 46

iatrogenicity 2
idiopathic hypersomnolence 67
ilioinguinal neuralgia 162
immobility 2
immune deficiency 3
impaired hearing 3
impaired vision 3
impecunity 3
impotence 3
inanition 3
incontinence 2
    faecal 136, 137
    urine 137–40
        containment methods 140
        drug therapy for 234
        incidence 137

investigations for 138
management 139
overflow 139
patterns of 137
stress 139
urge 139
infections 3, 140–2
fever and 94–7
general 140, 141
urinary 141, 142
informed consent, *see* consent
inhaled steroids 233
insanity 2
insomnia 3, 64
management approaches 65
treatments 66
instability 2
internal herniations of brain 72
intertrigo 185
intestinal obstruction 211
investigation, golden rules of 4
iron supplements 235
irritable colon 3
ischaemia, vertebrobasilar 100, 101
isolation 3
isosthenuria 53
itch 142–4
causes of 142, 143
clinical assessment of 143, 144
scabies 144
with rash 144

jaundice, description 37
joint disease,
pain in hand and wrist 172
pain in knee 175

ketoacidosis, diabetic 84
kidney disease, *see* renal disease
knee pain, *see* pain

L-dopa for Parkinsonism 238
labyrinthitis, acute 111
lamotrigine use in epilepsy 241
laxatives 244
legal aspects of treating mentally ill 19
legs,
basic physical examination 13
signs of disease in 16
ulcers of 186
leucocytosis 33
eosinophilia 35

lymphocytosis 35
monocytosis 35
neutrophilia 34
leukotriene receptor antagonists 233
lichenoid drug eruptions 185
lipids 29
assessment 30
management 30
liver function tests,
albumin 37
alkaline phosphatase 38
bilirubin 37
γ-glutamyl transpeptidase 38
generally used tests 36, 37
transaminases 38
locked-in syndrome 75
Loeb's Law 7
lung, shadows on 209
lymphocytosis 35

macrocytic anaemia 33
malignant/accelerated hypertension
132
management,
at end of life 25
golden rules of 6
of demented patient,
capacity 24
consent 21–4
of problems cf diagnosis 7
treatment cf care 25, 26
medical examination,
basic 9
basic physical examination 13
characteristic smells 14
for anaemia 32
for back pain 164
for cough 78
for funny turns 107
for headache 118
for hypertension 129
for incontinence 138
for movement disorders 197
gait and balance assessment 18
general neurological examination
249, 250
how to do a rectal examination 56
in abdominal pain 160
in patient with fever 96
of acutely breathless patient 57
of neck pain 178
of serious chest pain 168

of unconscious patient 69–71
medical history,
    anaemia questions 31
    for back pain 163
    for headache 117
    for movement disorders 197
    in abdominal pain 160
    methods of 9
    of cough 78
    of funny turns 107
    of neck pain 178
    of serious chest pain 168
    pointers to cause of coma from
        73
    suggested questions by system 12
    suggested questions on function 10,
        11
    what does the patient mean 97
medication headache 121
Menière's disease 110
meningitis 118
Mental Capacity Act 25
Mental Health Act 23
mental illness, legal aspects of treating
    medical conditions in 19
metformin 237
methicillin-resistant *Staphylococcus
    aureus* (MRSA), management of
    infection 97
microcytic anaemia 33
microsleeps 64
monocytosis 35
morbilliform eruptions 184
mouth,
    basic physical examination 13
    signs of disease in 14, 15
movement disorders 197–9
MRSA, management of infection
    97
multiple sensory impairments 110
musculoskeletal problems, questions
    on for medical history 12
myoclonic seizures 103
myoclonus, examination for 19
myxoedema coma 49

narcolepsy 67
nausea 144–6
    antiemetics for 146
    causes of 145
nebuliser therapy 60
neck,

basic physical examination, 14
bruits, basic physical examination
    13
pain, *see* pain
nefopam use in pain 154
nephritic syndrome 53
nephrotic syndrome 53
neuralgia,
    genitofemoral 162
    ilioinguinal 162
    post-herpetic 121
    temporomandibular 121
    trigeminal 120
neuroleptic drugs 198
neurological examination 18, 249, 250
    in dementia 19
neurology, questions on for medical
    history 12
neuroma, acoustic 111
neuropathy,
    entrapment 173
    examination for 19
    in calf 167
neutrophilia 34
neutrophils, causes of raised count 34
nicorandil for cardiovascular disease
    226
nitrates, for cardiovascular disease 225
non-steroidal anti-inflammatory agents
    153, 230, 231
normocytic anaemia 33
nosebleeds 146, 147
nutrition,
    feeding 195, 196
    in elderly diabetics 85
    iron supplements 235
    nutritional supplements 236
    swallowing problems 193
    vitamin supplements 235
    weight loss and 200–3

obstructive sleep apnoea 67
obstructive uropathy 53
oculocephalic responses 71
oedema, as a sign of disease 16
opioid analgesics 229, 230
    strong 155
    use in pain 154
    weak 155
opisthotonos 72
optokinetic eye movements 91
orexin deficiency 61

osmotic laxatives 244
osteoarthritis and knee pain 175
ototoxic drugs 110, 111
overflow incontinence 139
oxcarbazepine, use in epilepsy 240
oxygen therapy,
   compliance problems in dementia
      60
   in acute illness 59
   in chronic illness 59
   long-term 59

Paget's disease of the bone and hypercalcaemia 28
pain 147–81
   abdominal pain,
      acute 158
         causes of 158
      chronic 159
         causes of 159
      clinical history 160
      examination of 160
      gastro-oesophageal reflux dis-
         ease 161
      genitofemoral neuralgia 162
      ilioinguinal neuralgia 162
      peptic ulcer disease 161, 242
      sudden onset 206–8
   acute vs. chronic 150
   alternative drugs for 157
   analgesics used in 228
   anticonvulsants for 156
   antidepressants for 156
   aspirin for 228
   back (spine) pain 162–4
      causes of 162, 163
      history of 163
      lumbar spine 162
      management 164
      medical examination 164
   calf 165–7
      causes 165
      cellulitis 165
      deep vein thrombosis 166
      muscle cramp 165
      muscle injury 165
      neuropathy 167
      peripheral vascular disease 166
   chemicals/neurotransmitters
      involved in 149
   chest 167–70
      causes of 167

      investigations 169
      less serious 169
      management 169
      very serious 168
         medical examination 168
         medical history 168
   everywhere 170–2
      approach for 170
      causes of 171
   hand and wrist 172–4
      approach for 174
      causes of 173
      entrapment neuropathy 173
      joint disease 172
      management 174
   in demented patient with rectal
      cancer 209
   in rheumatoid arthritis with depres-
      sion 210
   knee 175
      causes of 175
      localised causes 177
      osteoarthritis 175
      rheumatoid disease 176
      septic arthritis 176
   mechanisms of 149
   modulation by central nervous sys-
      tem 149
   neck 177–9
      examination of 178
      history of 178
      management 179
      with neurological findings 177
      without neurological findings
         177
   nefopam for 154
   neuroanatomy of 148
   non-steroidal anti-inflammatory
      agents 153, 230, 231
   opioid analgesics for 154, 229, 230
   paracetamol for 152, 228
   shoulder 179, 180
      assessment 180
      causes of 179
      management 180
   treatment of 151, 152
palliative care 180, 181
paracetamol 228
   use in pain 152
parasomnias 66
Parkinsonism,
   antimuscarinic drugs for 239

dopamine agonists for 238
gait changes in 114
L-dopa for 238
psychiatric treatments and mobility maintenance 212
tremor and gait problems in 198
partial seizures 103, 104
patient education in diabetes mellitus 82
Patient's Charter 20
peptic ulcer disease 161, 242
perilymphatic fistula 111
peripheral vascular disease 166
pharmacodynamics 217
pharmacokinetics 216
phenobarbitone use in epilepsy 241
phenytoin use in epilepsy 241
phosphate and calcium abnormalities 28
phosphodiesterase inhibitors for cardiovascular disease 227
photosensitivity 185
platelets,
    abnormalities of 40
    increased production 40
    reduced production 40
pneumonia, hospital-acquired 245
post-herpetic neuralgia 121
postural hypotension 134, 135
posture and consciousness level 72
potassium, abnormalities of 41
prescribing,
    golden rules of 6
    guidelines for 215
    improving 218
    in elderly 215
    risk vs. benefit of drugs 217
pressure ulcers 187
presyncope 106
primary orthostatic tremor 199
primary prevention, of hyperlipidaemia 30
progressive supranuclear palsy 115
prolapse, uterovaginal 117
prostate disease,
    benign prostatic hypertrophy 55
    rectal examination technique 56, 57
proton pump inhibitors 243
proxy, role in Adults with Incapacity (Scotland) Act 2000
pruritus 142, 143

pseudo-silent presentation 3
pulse, basic physical examination 13

rashes 181–90
    actinic keratoses 182
    asteatotic dermatitis 182
    basal cell carcinoma 183
    blistering diseases 183
    causes of 181
    cellulitis 183
    contact dermatitis 184
    drug eruptions 184
    erythema multiforme 185
    fixed drug eruptions 185
    intertrigo 185
    leg ulcers 186
    lichenoid drug eruptions 185
    photosensitivity 185
    pressure ulcers 187
    rosacea 188
    scabies 188
    seborrhoeic dermatitis 188
    senile purpura 189
    shingles 189
    squamous carcinoma 189
    with itch 144
Raynaud's syndrome 173
rectal cancer 209
rectal examination technique 56, 57
rectum, bleeding from 190, 191
recurrent headache 119
refusal of treatment 211
renal disease,
    causes of kidney failure 52
    description 51
renal failure,
    acute 52
    chronic 53
    hypercalcaemia and 28
respiratory problems,
    β_2-agonists for 232
    antimuscarinic bronchodilators for 232
    cromoglycate for 233
    inhaled steroids for 233
    leukotriene receptor antagonists for 233
    questions on for medical history 12
reticular activating system 61
rheumatoid arthritis,
    depression and 210
    knee pain and 176

rights of patient 20
    Human Rights Act 20
    Patient's Charter 20
risk and consent 22
Romberg test 18
rosacea 188

saccadic eye movements 90
sarcoid and hypercalcaemia 28
scabies 144, 188
screening tests, suitable investigations 5
seborrhoeic dermatitis 188
seizures,
    absence 103, 240
    atonic 103
    classification of 102
    description 102
    generalised 240
    management of 104, 105
    myoclonic 103
    partial 103, 104, 240
    tonic 103
    tonic–clonic 103, 240
semethicone 243
senile purpura 189
septic arthritis and knee pain 176
shingles 189
shoulder pain, see pain
sight, see vision
silent presentation 2
singultus 127
skin,
    questions on for medical history 12
    rashes 181–90
    see also itch
sleep 60
    amount needed 63
    cf anaesthesia or coma 63
    cf blackouts 99
    microsleeps 64
    requirements for 62, 63
    stages of 62
sleep apnoea,
    central 67
    obstructive 67
sleep disorders,
    hypersomnias 67
    insomnias 64–6
    parasomnias 66
smooth pursuit eye movements 90
sodium,

abnormalities of 44
    metabolism of 44, 45
    renal handling of 44
somatosensory system 92
squamous carcinoma 189
statins,
    for cardiovascular disease 227
    use in hypertension 130
steroids, inhaled 233
stress incontinence 139
stridor 58
stroke 191, 192
    incidence 191
    management 192
stupor 67
subarachnoid haemorrhage 119
subcortical changes in gait 115
sulphonylureas 236
swallowing,
    feeding problems in dementia 194
    investigation of 194
    making feeding safer 195
    physiology 193
    problems with 193
    treatment of problems 195
syphilis serology, for diagnosis 5

temporal arteritis 119
temporomandibular neuralgia 121
tension pneumothorax 59
tension-type headache 120
thiazide diuretics and hypercalcaemia 28
thorax, signs of disease in 15
thrombosis, deep vein 166
thyroid disease,
    diagnosis in elderly 49
    Hashimoto's encephalopathy 51
    hyperthyroidism 50
    hypothyroidism 49
thyroid function tests, for diagnosis 5
thyroid hormones,
    abnormalities in 48
    in treatment of hypothyroidism 237
    metabolism of 49
thyroid-stimulating hormone 48
thyrotoxicosis and hypercalcaemia 28
thyrotropin-releasing hormone 48
tic douloureux 120
tiredness with weight loss in depression 205

tonic seizures 103
tonic–clonic seizures 103, 240
transaminases 38
transient ischaemic attacks 191
tremor 197–9
    cerebellar 199
    essential 198
    neuroleptic drugs and 198
    primary orthostatic 199
trigeminal neuralgia 120
tuberculosis 209
typical presentation 2

ulcers,
    as a sign of disease 16
    gastrointestinal, treatments for 242
    leg 186
    pressure 187
unconsciousness, *see* consciousness
uraemia 52
urea,
    and calcium abnormalities 28
    in acute renal failure 52
    in heart failure 126
    renal disease and 51
urge incontinence 139
urinary infections 141, 142, 245
    treatments 142
urinary retention, drug therapy for
    234
urine incontinence 137–40
urine stick testing, for diagnosis 5
urogenital problems, questions on for
    medical history 12
urticarial eruptions 184
uterovaginal prolapse 117
vaginal discharge 117

valproate, use in epilepsy 242
Valsalva manoeuvre 107, 108
varicella zoster virus 189
vascular disease, peripheral 166
vertebrobasilar insufficiency 100, 101
vertebrobasilar ischaemia 100, 101
vertigo 106
    benign paroxysmal positional 109
    post-concussional 111
vestibulo-ocular system interactions 91
vision,
    basic physical examination 13
    role in balance,
        optokinetic eye movements 91
        saccadic eye movements 90
        smooth pursuit eye movements
          90
    signs of disease in 15
vitamin supplements 235
vomiting 144–6
    antiemetics for 146
    causes of 145, 146
    mechanism 144
vulval disorders 116, 117

weight loss 200–3
    causes of 201, 202
    in depression 205
    investigations for 201
    treatment 203
white cell count, normal 34
withdrawal of artificial nutrition and
    hydration 26
wrist pain, *see* pain

vitamin B_{12}, for diagnosis 5